Interventional Ultrasound

Editor

DAVID L. WALDMAN

ULTRASOUND CLINICS

www.ultrasound.theclinics.com

Consulting Editor
VIKRAM DOGRA

April 2013 • Volume 8 • Number 2

ELSEVIER

1600 John F. Kennedy Boulevard • Suite 1800 • Philadelphia, Pennsylvania, 19103-2899

http://www.theclinics.com

ULTRASOUND CLINICS Volume 8, Number 2
April 2013 ISSN 1556-858X, ISBN-13: 978-1-4557-7342-8

Editor: Donald Mumford

Ultrasound Clinics (ISSN 1556-858X) is published quarterly by W.B. Saunders, 360 Park Avenue South, New York, NY 10010-1710. Months of publication are January, April, July, and October. Business and editorial offices: 1600 John F. Kennedy Boulevard, Suite 1800, Philadelphia, Pennsylvania 19103-2899. Accounting and circulation offices: 6277 Sea Harbor Drive, Orlando, FL 32887-4800. Periodicals postage paid at New York, NY, and additional mailing offices. Subscription prices are $258 per year for (US individuals), $309 per year for (US institutions), $123 per year for (US students and residents), $289 per year for (Canadian individuals), $345 per year for (Canadian institutions), $308 per year for (international individuals), $345 per year for (international institutions), and $147 per year for (Canadian and foreign students/residents). To receive student/resident rate, orders must be accompanied by name of affiliated institution, date of term, and the signature of program/residency coordinator on institution letterhead. Orders will be billed at individual rate until proof of status is received. Foreign air speed delivery is included in all Clinics subscription prices. All prices are subject to change without notice. **POSTMASTER:** Send address changes to *Ultrasound Clinics,* Elsevier Health Sciences Division, Subscription Customer Service, 3251 Riverport Lane, Maryland Heights, MO 63043. **Customer Service (orders, claims, online, change of address): Telephone: 1-800-654-2452 (U.S. and Canada); 314-447-8871 (outside U.S. and Canada). Fax: 314-447-8029. E-mail: journalscustomerservice-usa@elsevier.com (for print support); journalsonlinesupport-usa@elsevier.com (for online support).**

Reprints: For copies of 100 or more, of articles in this publication, please contact the Commercial Reprints Department, Elsevier Inc., 360 Park Avenue South, New York, NY 10010-1710. Tel.: (+1) 212-633-3812; Fax: (+1) 212-462-1935; E-mail: reprints@elsevier.com.

Printed and bound by CPI Group (UK) Ltd, Croydon, CR0 4YY
Transferred to Digital Printing, 2013

Contributors

CONSULTING EDITOR

VIKRAM DOGRA, MD
Professor of Radiology, Urology, and
Biomedical Engineering, Director of Ultrasound
and Associate Chair for Education and
Research, Department of Imaging Sciences,
University of Rochester School of Medicine
and Dentistry, Rochester, New York

EDITOR

DAVID L. WALDMAN, MD, PhD, FACR, FSIR
Professor and Chairman, Department of
Imaging Sciences, School of Medicine and
Dentistry, University of Rochester Medical
Center, Rochester, New York

AUTHORS

JEAN-FRANCOIS AUBRY, PhD
Department of Neurosurgery, Radiation
Oncology, The University of Virginia School
of Medicine, Charlottesville, Virginia; Institut
Langevin, ESPCI, Paris, France

WILLIAM P. BREHMER, MD
Radiology Resident, Division of Vascular
Interventional Radiology, Department of
Imaging sciences, University of Virginia Health
System, Charlottesville, Virginia

DEVANG BUTANI, MD
Assistant Professor, Division of Interventional
Radiology, Department of Imaging Sciences,
University of Rochester Medical Center,
Rochester, New York

NANCY CARSON, MBA, RDMS, RVT
Department of Imaging Sciences, University
of Rochester Medical Center, Rochester,
New York

SHIRLEY CHAN, MD
Radiology Resident, PGY 3, Department of
Imaging Sciences, University of Rochester
Medical Center, Rochester, New York

DESI DENNIS, MD
Section of Vascular and Interventional
Radiology, Mallinckrodt Institute of Radiology,
Washington University, St Louis, Missouri

DOUGLAS DRUMSTA, MD
Resident of Radiology, Department of Imaging
Sciences, University of Rochester, Rochester,
New York

JEREMY B. DUDA, MD
Chief Radiology Resident, Department of
Imaging Sciences, University of Rochester
Medical Center, Rochester, New York

ADAM S. FANG, MD
Department of Imaging Sciences, University
of Rochester Medical Center, Rochester,
New York

ARIK HANANEL, MD, MBA, BsCS
Visiting Assistant Professor of Research,
Department of Radiation Oncology, The
University of Virginia School of Medicine;
Scientific and Medical Director, Focused
Ultrasound Surgery Foundation,
Charlottesville, Virginia

TRAVIS J. HILLEN, MD
Assistant Professor in Radiology,
Musculoskeletal Section, Mallinckrodt Institute
of Radiology, Washington University School of
Medicine in St. Louis, St Louis, Missouri

GEORGE A. HOLLAND, MD
Associate Professor, Department of Imaging
Sciences, University of Rochester Medical
Center, Rochester, New York

ABID IRSHAD, MD
Professor of Radiology, Director of Breast
Imaging, Department of Radiology and
Radiological Science, Medical University of
South Carolina, Charleston, South Carolina

JACK JENNINGS, MD
Assistant Professor in Radiology,
Musculoskeletal Section, Mallinckrodt Institute
of Radiology, Washington University School of
Medicine in St. Louis, St Louis, Missouri

KATHERINE KAPROTH-JOSLIN, MD, PhD
Resident of Radiology, Department of Imaging
Sciences, University of Rochester, Rochester,
New York

VALERIY KHEYFITS, MD
Assistant Professor, Department of Imaging
Sciences, University of Rochester Medical
Center, Rochester, New York

DAVID E. LEE, MD
Associate Professor of Imaging Sciences,
University of Rochester Medical Center,
University of Rochester, Rochester, New York

JESSICA LEE, MD
Interventional Radiology Fellow, Mallinckrodt
Institute of Radiology, St Louis, Missouri

THOMAS LOSTRACCO, MD
Section of Interventional Radiology, Department
of Imaging Sciences, University of Rochester
Medical Center, Rochester, New York

EDWARD J. MATHES, PA-C
Staff Physician Assistant, Division of Vascular
and Interventional Radiology, Department of
Imaging Sciences, Strong Memorial Hospital;
Associate Clinical Professor, Physician
Assistant Program, Rochester Institute of
Technology, Rochester, New York

JOHN MCGRATH, MD
Department of Radiology, University of
Rochester Medical Center, Rochester,
New York

OLEG MIRONOV, MD
2nd Year Radiology Resident, Department of
Imaging Sciences, University of Rochester
Medical Center, Rochester, New York

MEENA K. MOORTHY, MD, MBA
Musculoskeletal Radiology Fellow,
Department of Imaging Sciences, University
of Rochester Medical Center, Rochester,
New York

MIKE S. NGUYEN, MD
Resident, Department of Imaging Sciences,
University of Rochester Medical Center,
Rochester, New York

REFKY NICOLA, MS, DO
Section of Interventional Radiology,
Department of Imaging Sciences, University
of Rochester Medical Center, Rochester,
New York

AVICE M. O'CONNELL, MD, FACR
Director of Women's Imaging, Professor of
Clinical Imaging Sciences, Department of
Imaging Sciences, University of Rochester
Medical Center, Rochester, New York

JOSEPH REIS, MD
Radiology Resident (R-4), Department of
Imaging Sciences, University of Rochester
Medical Center, Rochester, New York

DEBORAH J. RUBENS, MD
Professor and Associate Chair of Imaging
Sciences, University of Rochester Medical
Center, University of Rochester, Rochester,
New York

NAEL SAAD, MD
Assistant Professor of Radiology and Surgery,
Mallinckrodt Institute of Radiology,
Washington University, St Louis, Missouri

WAEL E. SAAD, MD, FSIR
Professor of Radiology, Division of Vascular
Interventional Radiology, Department of
Imaging sciences, University of Virginia Health
System, Charlottesville, Virginia

TALIA SASSON, MD
Department of Imaging Sciences, University of Rochester Medical Center, Rochester, New York

ASHWANI K. SHARMA, MD
Assistant Professor of Imaging Sciences, Interventional Radiology, University of Rochester Medical Center, University of Rochester, Rochester, New York

DAVID N. SIEGEL, MD, FSIR
Chief, Division of Vascular/Interventional Radiology, North Shore Long Island Jewish Health System, New Hyde Park, New York

LABIB SYED, MD, MPH
Section of Interventional Radiology, Department of Imaging Sciences, University of Rochester Medical Center, Rochester, New York

DAVID L. WALDMAN, MD, PhD, FACR, FSIR
Professor and Chairman, Department of Imaging Sciences, School of Medicine and Dentistry, University of Rochester Medical Center, Rochester, New York

SUSAN VOCI, MD
Department of Imaging Sciences, University of Rochester Medical Center, Rochester, New York

Contributors

TALIA SASSON, MD
Department of Imaging Sciences, University of Rochester Medical Center, Rochester, New York

ASHWANI K. SHARMA, MD
Assistant Professor of Imaging Sciences, Interventional Radiology, University of Rochester Medical Center, University of Rochester, Rochester, New York

DAVID N. SIEGEL, MD, FSIR
Chief, Division of Vascular/Interventional Radiology, North Shore Long Island Jewish Health System, New Hyde Park, New York

LABIB SYED, MD, MPH
Section of Interventional Radiology, Department of Imaging Sciences, University of Rochester Medical Center, Rochester, New York

DAVID L. WALDMAN, MD, PhD, FACR, FSIR
Professor and Chairman, Department of Imaging Sciences, School of Medicine and Dentistry, University of Rochester Medical Center, Rochester, New York

SUSAN VOCI, MD
Department of Imaging Sciences, University of Rochester Medical Center, Rochester, New York

Contents

platforms. These improvements make IVUS a valuable tool and adjunct to conventional angiography in endovascular interventions. Whereas conventional angiography enables visualization of the caliber and contour of a vessel lumen, IVUS enables accurate visualization of vessel wall anatomy as well as adjacent structures and therefore provides important diagnostic information and clinical utility in endovascular interventions, especially in the setting of complex anatomy that is unclear on angiography.

ULTRASOUND CLINICS

DOWNLOAD
Free App!

Review Articles
THE CLINICS

NOW AVAILABLE FOR YOUR iPhone and iPad

PROGRAM OBJECTIVE:

The goal of the *Ultrasound Clinics* is to keep practicing radiologists and radiology residents up to date with current clinical practice in ultrasound by providing timely articles reviewing the state of the art in patient care.

TARGET AUDIENCE

Practicing radiologists, radiology residents and other healthcare professionals who provide care based on radiologic findings.

LEARNING OBJECTIVES

Upon completion of this activity, participants will be able to:

1. Review the role of ultrasound in the postoperative evaluation, maturation process, and postoperative evaluation of hemodialysis access.
2. Describe ultrasound-guided superficial structures biopsy and solid organ biopsy.
3. Utilize the use of ultrasound in musculoskeletal interventions and duplex ultrasound in the management of varicose veins.

ACCREDITATION

The Elsevier Office of Continuing Medical Education (EOCME) is accredited by the Accreditation Council for Continuing Medical Education (ACCME) to provide continuing medical education for physicians.

The EOCME designates this journal-based CME activity for a maximum of 15 *AMA PRA Category 1 Credit*(s)™. Physicians should claim only the credit commensurate with the extent of their participation in the activity.

All other health care professionals completing continuing education credit for this activity will be issued a certificate of participation.

DISCLOSURE OF CONFLICTS OF INTEREST

The EOCME assesses conflict of interest with its instructors, faculty, planners, and other individuals who are in a position to control the content of CME activities. All relevant conflicts of interest that are identified are thoroughly vetted by EOCME for fair balance, scientific objectivity, and patient care recommendations. EOCME is committed to providing its learners with CME activities that promote improvements or quality in healthcare and not a specific proprietary business or a commercial interest.

The planning committee, staff, authors and editors listed below have identified no financial relationships or relationships to products or devices they or their spouse/life partner have with commercial interest related to the content of this CME activity:
Jean Francois Aubry, PhD; William Brehmer, MD; Devang Butani, MD; Nancy Carson, MBA; Shirley Chan, MD; Mahendra Kumar Chandran; Desi Dennis; Douglas Drumsta, MD; Jeremy Duda, MD; Adam Fang, MD; George Holland, MD; Abid Irshad; Katherine Kaproth-Joslin, MD; Valeriy Kheyfits, MD; Sandy Lavery; David E. Lee, MD; Jessica Lee, MD; Thomas LoStracco, MD; Edward Mathes, PA; John McGrath, MD; Jill McNair; Oleg Mironov, MD; Meena Moorthy, MD, MBA; Mike Nguyen, MD; Refky Nicola, DO; Avice O'Connell, MD; Joseph Reis, MD; Deborah J. Rubens, MD; Nael Saad, MD; Talia Sasson, MD; Ashwani K. Sharma, MD; Gretchen Spencer; Labib Syed, MD; Susan Voci, MD; and David L. Waldman, MD.

The planning committee, staff, authors and editors listed below have identified financial relationships or relationships to products or devices they or their spouse/life partner have with commercial interest related to the content of this CME activity:
Arik Hananel, MD, MBA has stock ownership in InSightec.
Travis J. Hillen, MD is a consultant for Biomedical Systems and OnControl.
Jack Jennings, MD is a consultant/advisor and on the speaker's bureau for Dfine Inc.
Wael E. Saad, MD is a consultant for Boston Scientific; is on the speaker's bureau for Atrium; and has received a research grant from Siemens.
David N. Siegel, MD is on speaker's bureau for Celonova Bioscience and Philips Medical Systems; and is a consultant/advisor for Celonova Bioscience, Boston Scientific and Medtronic Corp.

UNAPPROVED/OFF-LABEL USE DISCLOSURE

The EOCME requires CME faculty to disclose to the participants:

1. When products or procedures being discussed are off-label, unlabelled, experimental, and/or investigational (not US Food and Drug Administration (FDA) approved); and
2. Any limitations on the information presented, such as data that are preliminary or that represent ongoing research, interim analyses, and/or unsupported opinions. Faculty may discuss information about pharmaceutical agents that is outside of FDA-approved labelling. This information is intended solely for CME and is not intended to promote off-label use of these medications. If you have any questions, contact the medical affairs department of the manufacturer for the most recent prescribing information.

TO ENROLL

To enroll in the *Ultrasounds Clinic* Continuing Medical Education program, call customer service at 1-800-654-2452 or sign up online at http://www.theclinics.com/home/cme. The CME program is available to subscribers for an additional annual fee of USD 212.

METHOD OF PARTICIPATION

In order to claim credit, participants must complete the following:

1. Complete enrolment as indicated above.
2. Read the activity.
3. Complete the CME Test and Evaluation. Participants must achieve a score of 70% on the test. All CME Tests and Evaluations must be completed online.

CME INQUIRIES/SPECIAL NEEDS

For all CME inquiries or special needs, please contact elsevierCME@elsevier.com.

Preface

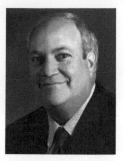

David L. Waldman, MD, PhD, FACR, FSIR
Editor

Ultrasound Clinics is a publication devoted to medical ultrasound. This quarterly journal is a welcome addition to the demand for up-to-date knowledge on imaging involving every aspect of sonography. This issue is devoted to the use of ultrasound in the practice of Vascular and Interventional Radiology.

With advances in modern imaging systems, practicing physicians have a wide array of diagnostic tools at their fingertips. Ultrasound is quickly becoming one of the mainstays of diagnostic medicine. Ultrasound techniques have improved with new materials, faster computer processing, and the use of high-frequency ultrasound for therapy. Newer techniques in image registration allow real-time imaging scanning over static images from modalities, including CT and MRI, which allows the interventional radiologist to go beyond traditional interventional procedures.

Topics in this issue have been chosen with particular attention to the tools and techniques of Vascular and Interventional Radiology. We have recruited Interventional Radiologists and Ultrasound physicians from all over the country. It is my hope that the key concepts will benefit readers in the practice of both Vascular and Interventional Radiology and Ultrasound.

I'm honored to be the guest editor of this issue of the *Ultrasound Clinics*. My sincerest thanks to Patty Miller for helping me assemble this edition.

This edition is dedicated to our colleague and my friend, Larry Sahler, MD, who passed away suddenly during the summer of 2012. He was an outstanding Interventional Radiologist and typified the mantra of innovation.

David L. Waldman, MD, PhD, FACR, FSIR
Department of Imaging Sciences
University of Rochester Medical Center
School of Medicine and Dentistry
601 Elmwood Avenue, Box 648
Rochester, NY 14642, USA

E-mail address:
David_Waldman@URMC.Rochester.edu

Ultrasound Clin 8 (2013) xiii
http://dx.doi.org/10.1016/j.cult.2013.01.001
1556-858X/13/$ – see front matter © 2013 Published by Elsevier Inc.

Breast Ultrasonography

Avice M. O'Connell, MD[a],*, Abid Irshad, MD[b],
Mike S. Nguyen, MD[a]

KEYWORDS

• Ultrasound • Breast • Screening • Intervention • Elastography • Automated • Contrast-Enhanced

KEY POINTS

- Screening breast ultrasonography is becoming more widespread, and recent legislation in several states has led to supplemental screening for women with dense breasts on mammography.
- Targeted or diagnostic ultrasonography is invaluable in the workup of mammographic and magnetic resonance imaging findings.
- Ultrasound-guided interventions such as preoperative needle localizations and biopsies are in the mainstream of breast imaging.

 Videos of breast biopsy techniques accompany this article

SURVEILLANCE, DIAGNOSIS, AND INTERVENTION: THE NEXT GENERATION

Introduction

The role of ultrasound (US) in breast imaging dates back several decades to the late 1970s, when US was limited to the distinction of solid from cystic masses. Technical advances have given dedicated breast US an invaluable role in diagnosis and intervention for many breast conditions, and increasingly as a supplement for screening. US is in many respects the ideal modality for breast imaging: widely available, relatively inexpensive, pain free, and there is no ionizing radiation or intravenous contrast.

However, many issues exist that make US less than ideal for the detection of early breast cancer. The most significant drawback is the high number of false-positive findings (cysts and fibrocystic clusters, fibroadenoma, papillomas, fat lobules, and fat necrosis), leading to a high percentage of negative biopsies.[1] Training is an issue with respect to reliability and reproducibility, whether the physician, technologist, or automated whole-breast US machine performs the examination.

According to the ACRIN 6666 (American College of Radiology Imaging Network 6666) study, it takes a physician approximately 20 minutes to perform a full bilateral examination. Radiologists do not have time to scan every screening patient.

Screening Breast US

Women with dense breasts, greater than 50%, are 2 to 6 times more likely to develop breast cancer, which is independent of the lower sensitivity of mammography in dense breasts (**Fig. 1**).[2] The lay public has increasing awareness of the increased risk with dense breasts. Both the American College of Radiology and Society of Breast Imaging have addressed recommendations for breast cancer screening.[3] Both groups suggest that US may have a role in supplemental screening for women with mammographically dense breast parenchyma after conventional 2-view mammogram, in which masses and other abnormalities may be obscured.

The lack of specificity for US findings was shown by the ACRIN 6666 study, which involved women with dense breasts and increased high risk of breast cancer. There were 4.2 additional cancers

[a] Department of Imaging Sciences, University of Rochester Medical Center, 601 Elmwood Avenue, Box 648, Rochester, NY 14642, USA; [b] Department of Radiology and Radiological Science, Medical University of South Carolina, 169 Ashley Avenue, Charleston, SC 29425, USA
* Corresponding author.
E-mail address: Avice_Oconnell@urmc.rochester.edu

Ultrasound Clin 8 (2013) 109–116
http://dx.doi.org/10.1016/j.cult.2012.12.001
1556-858X/13/$ – see front matter © 2013 Elsevier Inc. All rights reserved.

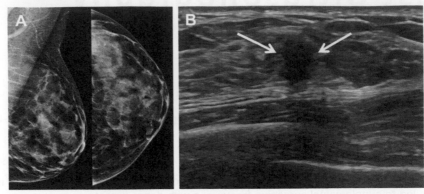

Fig. 1. Dense breast. (*A*) Craniocaudal and mediolateral-oblique view mammogram of the left breast, which is essentially negative. The breast parenchyma is heterogeneously dense which lowers the sensitivity of mammogram. (*B*) US image of the left breast, showing a small infiltrative ductal carcinoma (*arrows*), which was node negative at diagnosis.

per 1000 women (28% more) after an experienced physician mammographer performed whole-breast US in addition to standard mammography. The downside was the high false-positive results. There were 4 times as many false-positive biopsies compared with mammography alone. All cancers were small and node negative.

As of December 2012, five states (Connecticut [2009], Texas [2011], Virginia [2012], California [2012], and New York [2012]) have passed breast density laws that mandate notifying all women of their breast density in the summary report sent with their mammogram results and recommendations. Despite good intentions, these laws create more confusion and anxiety unless insurance companies agree to cover screening US.

A study encompassing the first 3 years after passage of the Connecticut breast density law[4] shows that an additional 3.2 breast cancers per 1000 women screened were found by US and not seen on mammography. All were small (less than 1 cm), with a positive biopsy rate of 5.6%,

and the calculated cost per cancer diagnosed is $60,267 (based on US Medicare rates).

US in the Diagnostic Setting

US is invaluable in the workup of a palpable abnormality. The evaluation of any palpable mass or thickening is incomplete without targeted US directed at the abnormality. In the presence of a palpable mass, US must be performed to evaluate any palpable finding, even in the setting of a negative mammogram (**Fig. 2**). US can then be used to guide biopsy for tissue diagnosis and to assess for involved axillary lymph nodes.

Second-Look US After Positive Magnetic Resonance Imaging for Breast Cancer

Another recent use of breast US is in the diagnosis and management of women with newly diagnosed breast cancer. After breast magnetic resonance (MR) imaging, additional identified findings are evaluated using targeted second-look US (**Fig. 3**).

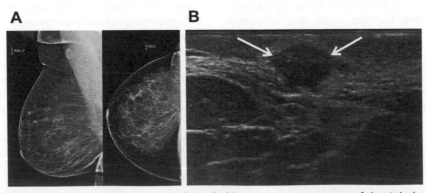

Fig. 2. Palpable mass. (*A*) Craniocaudal and mediolateral-oblique view mammogram of the right breast. Mammogram is negative and the parenchymal pattern is *not* dense. (*B*) US image of the palpable area showing a small cancer adjacent to the nipple (*arrows*).

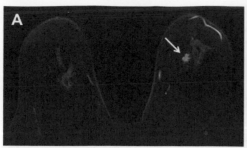 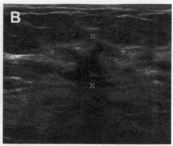

Fig. 3. (*A*) Breast MR imaging shows an irregular mass (*arrow*) seen in the left breast. (*B*) Targeted US image of the area in the left breast showing irregular suspicious mass (*calipers*), which can be easily biopsied under US guidance.

If the abnormalities are seen on US, a biopsy can be performed more easily and comfortably under US guidance.

FUTURE BREAST US TECHNOLOGIES
Introduction

Breast US is benefitting from new technologies that yield more information about breast lesions and that can lead to improved diagnosis and reduce the false-positive biopsy rate.

Elastography

Benign and malignant breast lesions can have overlapping morphologic features on US. In general, malignant lesions are commonly firmer than benign lesions. Elastography produces images based on tissue stiffness, which may help differentiate benign from malignant lesions. Two elasticity modes are available: compression elastography and shear wave elastography.

Compression elastography produces images based on tissue displacement and allows for the qualitative assessment of the lesions using an elastogram. Most companies use compression elastography to assess the relative stiffness between a lesion and the surrounding breast tissue (**Fig. 4**).[5]

Shear wave elastography is used to quantify the stiffness of the tissue by the use of a special push pulse, which creates a shear wave propagation through the tissue.[6] By measuring the velocity of the shear wave, tissue stiffness can be calculated. Shear wave elastography displays more quantitative information than free-hand elastography and can be used to characterize breast lesions.[5] A recent study showed that a higher mean stiffness value using shear wave elastography is associated with poorer prognosis. In the future, this finding may help with treatment planning.[7] Moreover, shear wave elastography is independent of the sonographer who performs the examination.

Although elastography has high sensitivities (70.1%–86.5%) and specificities (52%–95.7%)

for characterizing breast lesions as benign or malignant, studies have not consistently demonstrated improved diagnostic performance. This finding is true whether independent or in combination with B-mode ultrasonography.[8,9] Other limitations of elastography include large interobserver variation and significant time to perform the elastography examinations. Advances in elastography hardware and software may help to overcome these shortcomings. Elastography is a promising technology that may improve diagnostic performance and reduce the number of negative biopsies.

Automated Breast US

Mammography misses at least half of breast cancers in women with dense breasts. Most of these cancers are small and hence at a stage at which treatment is typically less invasive and has improved outcomes. Screening handheld US is often viewed as impractical because of the operator dependency, time requirements, and high false-positive results. The limitations of handheld sonography have led to the development of automated breast US (ABUS). The goal of ABUS is to produce standardized, reproducible diagnostic images while using automated US technology. Previously, the transducer frequency and overall quality of these machines were inferior to traditional handheld machines. Recent advances in ABUS technology have produced equivalent transducer frequencies.[9] Kelly and Richwald[10] reported that ABUS combined with screening mammography doubles the overall cancer detection rate and triples the number of invasive cancers 1 cm or less found in women with dense breasts.

Over the past half decade, 3 companies have introduced ABUS systems: SomoV (U-Systems, Silicon Valley, CA), Automated Whole Breast Ultrasound (AWBUS) (SonoCine, Reno, NV), and the ACUSON S2000 Automated Breast Volume Scanner (ABVS) (Siemens Healthcare, Reno, NV).

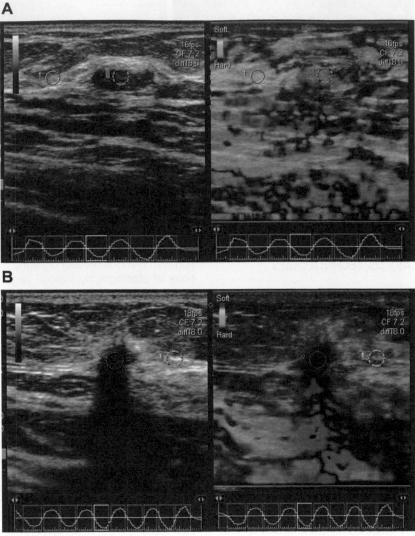

Fig. 4. Elastogram. (*A*) Gray-scale and elastogram image of a benign mass. The color map shows the mass (*pink circle*) to be in relatively soft range on the color scale. (*B*) A malignant mass (*pink circle*), which shows hard tissue on the elasticity color map.

In September 2012, the US Food and Drug Administration for the first time granted approval of an ABUS system for women with dense breasts.

Computer-Aided Diagnosis in US

Although computer-aided diagnosis (CAD) is clinically accepted in mammography, CAD is now being applied to US. Studies on sonographic CAD have shown improved sensitivity and specificity.[11] CAD is effective with both handheld sonography and the new ABUS.[12,13]

Fusion Imaging

Image registration involves the fusion of data from two or more modalities. The most widely used clinical application is positron emission tomography-computed tomography (PET/CT). Fusing real-time sonographic data with CT or MR imaging is still primarily investigational, but vendors have begun offering such capabilities in diverse fields as neurosurgery, prostate imaging, and abdominal biopsies.[9] This technology may lead to improved breast biopsy, localization, and treatment techniques.

Three-Dimensional Imaging

Three-dimensional (3D) breast sonography is not widely used. Although two-dimensional and 3D breast sonography are comparable in diagnostic performance, 3D sonography has the advantage of providing multiplanar information. Multiplanar information can aid in the characterization and documentation of breast lesions.[9] 3D imaging has the potential of being combined with other imaging technologies such as CAD, ABUS, and fusion imaging to improve sensitivity and specificity.

Contrast-Enhanced US

Contrast-enhanced US (CEUS) uses a microbubble or solid-particle contrast agent to delineate macro-circulation and microcirculation in a region of interest by increasing backscatter echoes. CEUS has found applications in areas such as liver and heart imaging and even drug and gene delivery.[14] Initial experiences with CEUS in breast imaging were disappointing, because it was not possible to differentiate between benign and malignant breast lesions.[15] Over the last decade, advances in US equipment, CEUS software, and the introduction of second-generation contrast agents have greatly improved the sensitivity and specificity of CEUS. Malignant lesions show early washin with increased enhancement and fast washout compared with benign lesions. However, there is no consensus regarding vascularization patterns to differentiate benign from malignant lesions.[15] Moreover, while ultrasound contrast agents can be used clinically in other countries like Canada, they have not yet been approved for clinical use by the US Food and Drug Administration. CEUS is another promising technology that may improve diagnostic performance and reduce the number of negative biopsies.

BREAST INTERVENTIONAL AND POSTINTERVENTION MANAGEMENT
Introduction

The BI-RADS (Breast Imaging Reporting and Data System) guidelines show that the threshold for obtaining a breast biopsy for a suspicious lesion is kept low (>2% chance of being malignant). Most of the solid masses that do not fulfill the criteria of a benign lesion and most of the complex cystic lesions need to be biopsied to exclude breast cancer.

The precautionary measures taken for a breast biopsy are generally not as stringent as those for biopsy of internal organs. A prebiopsy blood workup is generally not necessary. Because the breast is an easily compressible organ, excessive bleeding is rare from a breast biopsy. Although the anticoagulants may be stopped at an appropriate time before biopsy considering the risk versus benefit, some studies have shown no significant increased risk for bleeding in patients who are on anticoagulants compared with those who are off anticoagulants.[16,17] Certain measures such as using local anesthetic with epinephrine and compressing for a longer period after the biopsy may decrease the chances of excessive bleeding if biopsy is performed while the patient remains on anticoagulants.[16,17]

Diagnostic tissue sampling of breast lesions can be performed using various techniques such as core needle biopsy (CNB), fine-needle aspiration (FNA), stereotactic biopsy, and fluid aspiration from cystic lesions. The image-guided biopsies can be performed under US guidance, mammographic guidance, or MR imaging guidance, depending on which modality shows the lesion best. US-guided biopsy is the most commonly performed procedure for tissue diagnosis of breast masses.

Use of color Doppler is helpful in avoiding any large blood vessels in the needle path and selecting the appropriate site for needle insertion. In addition, color Doppler may show any hypervascular areas within the tumor that may be easily avoided during the biopsy to prevent excessive bleeding.

Core Needle Biopsy

US-guided core biopsy is usually performed using 11 to 16 gauge (G) needles. Various needles are being used in clinical practice with either spring-loaded or vacuum-assisted technology. Recently, there has been an increasing trend toward the use of vacuum-assisted and larger-gauge needles (usually 14 G or less). Biopsy needles are introduced under US guidance either using a free-hand technique or with the use of a coaxial-introducer system. Usually 3 to 8 samples are obtained during US biopsies, depending on the needle system used. Keeping the needle parallel to the chest wall is important, especially for deep lesions. Adequacy of sampling is best assessed on real-time imaging during the biopsy procedures. It is important to position the lesion within the area of the cutting notch. The cutting notch is proximal to the tip and the needles have a 5-mm to 6-mm noncutting dead space at the needle tip (**Fig. 5**). Inclusion of a little normal breast tissue in the biopsy samples is desirable, because it may increase the diagnostic accuracy of identifying the disease.

Recently, there has been an increased trend of placing a titanium clip marker at the site of biopsy. This marker serves as a guide for subsequent surgical excision in cases of cancer or high-risk lesions. In case of a benign result, the marker shows on the subsequent mammograms as an indicator of a previous benign biopsy. The placement of the marker is considered crucial in

A

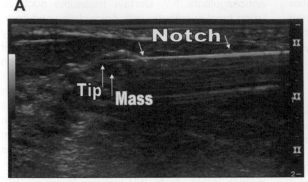

B

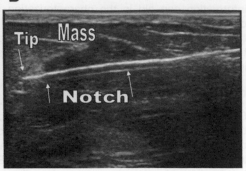

Fig. 5. Needle positioning. (*A*) Inadequate sampling of the mass (*arrows*). The portion of the needle within the mass mostly includes the dead space. The position of the cutting notch (*short arrows*) is proximal to the mass. (*B*) Adequate positioning of the lesion within the area of the cutting notch (*arrows*).

2 situations. First, in patients with newly diagnosed breast cancers that are to receive neoadjuvant therapy before lumpectomy. In some of these cases, the tumor may completely disappear, leaving the clip as the only guide for subsequent lumpectomy. Second, when the lesions/calcifications are so small that these may be completely removed during the biopsy procedure, placement of a clip ensures accurate subsequent surgical removal of the tissue, if warranted by subsequent pathologic diagnosis. Postclip placement mammograms are routinely obtained to confirm the position of the clip in relation to the lesion. Compared with stereotactic biopsy, clip displacement is less common in US-guided biopsy, possibly because of the accordion effect seen in the former.

Stereotactic biopsies are mostly performed for calcifications. However, in many situations when a mammographic density or mass is either not seen on US or has an uncertain correlation, a stereotactic biopsy may be the only way to obtain tissue sampling. Because generally only 15° angulations are used for needle positioning, lesions that are seen only on 1 view may also sometimes be amenable to a stereotactic biopsy.

Cyst Aspiration

Cystic lesions of the breast are frequently aspirated either for cytologic analysis of the fluid (in cases of lesions with suspicious US features) or for symptomatic relief of pain and discomfort (in cases of simple or complicated cysts). Many studies have shown extremely low risk of breast cancer in cysts from which nonhemorrhagic fluid is aspirated.[18–20] In current clinical practice in many institutions, the aspirated fluid is sent for cytology only if it has a hemorrhagic appearance and is otherwise discarded.

US-Guided Wire Localization

The lesions that are well seen on US can easily be localized by US-guided wire placement. The advantages of US-guided over mammographic-guided wire placement include no radiation, the ability to use the shortest route, and potentially quicker procedure. US guidance may still be preferable in many cases, even when a metallic biopsy clip has been placed during the initial biopsy. Especially for the masses that are well seen on US and less well seen on mammogram (usually in patients with dense breasts), US guidance ensures accurate wire placement through the lesion. On the other hand, mammographic localization of the clip in these patients with dense breasts may inadvertently leave the lesion behind if there has been an unnoticed clip displacement. A postwire-placement mammogram may be obtained to show the position of the mass or the clip. However, if the lesion is not well seen on the mammogram, the measurements of the wire may also be obtained on US (**Fig. 6**) and sent to the operating room for the surgeons.

Management of the Axilla

In routine practice, whenever a suspicious lesion is seen in the breast for which a biopsy would be recommended, axillary US should be performed at the same time. If abnormal lymph nodes are seen, a breast biopsy and axillary node biopsy/FNA can be performed at the same time. The criteria for an abnormal lymph node include loss of fatty hilum, compressed hilum, asymmetric cortical thickening, cortical nodularity, cortical thickness greater than fatty hilum, and abnormal nonhilar vascular supply to the lymph node. Some practices use cortical thickness greater than 3 to 5 mm as a cutoff for nodal biopsy in

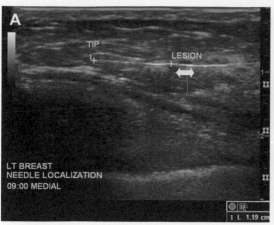 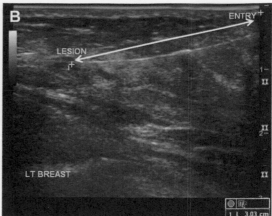

Fig. 6. Wire measurements on US. (*A*) Measurement of the wire from the lesion to the wire tip (*calipers*). (*B*) Distance (length) of the wire from the skin entry to the lesion.

patients who have cancer. Whereas some practices routinely perform a CNB for axillary nodes, others prefer FNA, which is safer and is frequently sufficient for making a diagnosis by the on-site pathologist. CNB in the axilla should be performed with care, because of the presence of adjacent vessels and nerves.

Postbiopsy management mainly depends on pathologic diagnosis and sampling confidence. Subsequent lumpectomy is performed in cases of malignancy either before or after neoadjuvant chemotherapy. In addition, certain high-risk pathologies such as atypical ductal hyperplasia, atypical lobular hyperplasia, and lobular carcinoma in situ, certain papillary neoplasms, or complex sclerosing lesions may also be surgically excised. The radiologic-pathologic concordance is made by the breast imagers, and the decision is made if the pathologic diagnosis explains the imaging appearance. Generally, all extremely suspicious (generally BI-RADS 5) lesions are subjected to surgical excision for a definite diagnosis in cases of discordant findings.

VIDEOS

Videos related to this article can be found online at http://dx.doi.org/10.1016/j.cult.2012.12.001.

REFERENCES

1. Berg WA, Cosgrove DO, Dore CJ, et al. Shear-wave elastography improves the specificity of breast US: the BE1 multinational study of 939 masses. Radiology 2012;262:435–49.
2. Harvey JA, Bovbjerg VE. Quantitative assessment of mammographic breast density: relationship with breast cancer risk. Radiology 2004;230:29–41.
3. Lee CH, Dershaw DD, Kopans D, et al. Breast cancer screening with imaging: recommendations from the Society of Breast Imaging and the ACR on the use of mammography, breast MRI, breast ultrasound, and other technologies for the detection of clinically occult breast cancer. J Am Coll Radiol 2010;7:18–27.
4. Hooley RJ, Greenberg KL, Stackhouse RM, et al. Screening US in patients with mammographically dense breasts: initial experience with Connecticut Public Act 09-41. Radiology 2012;265: 59–69.
5. Balleyguier C, Canale S, Ben Hassen W, et al. Breast elasticity: principles, technique, results: an update and overview of commercially available software. Eur J Radiol 2012. [Epub ahead of print].
6. Barr RG. Sonographic breast elastography: a primer. J Ultrasound Med 2012;31:773–83.
7. Evans A, Whelehan P, Thomson K, et al. Invasive breast cancer: relationship between shear-wave elastographic findings and histologic prognostic factors. Radiology 2012;263:673–7.
8. Sadigh G, Carlos RC, Neal CH, et al. Ultrasonographic differentiation of malignant from benign breast lesions: a meta-analytic comparison of elasticity and BIRADS scoring. Breast Cancer Res Treat 2012;133:23–35.
9. Hashimoto BE. New sonographic breast technologies. Semin Roentgenol 2011;46:292–301.
10. Kelly KM, Richwald GA. Automated whole-breast ultrasound: advancing the performance of breast cancer screening. Semin Ultrasound CT MR 2011; 32:273–80.
11. Weinstein SP, Conant EF, Sehgal C. Technical advances in breast ultrasound imaging. Semin Ultrasound CT MR 2006;27:273–83.
12. Moon WK, Shen YW, Huang CS, et al. Computer-aided diagnosis for the classification of breast

masses in automated whole breast ultrasound images. Ultrasound Med Biol 2011;37:539–48.

13. Shen WC, Chang RF, Moon WK, et al. Breast ultrasound computer-aided diagnosis using BI-RADS features. Acad Radiol 2007;14:928–39.

14. Xu HX. Contrast-enhanced ultrasound: the evolving applications. World J Radiol 2009;1:15–24.

15. Drudi FM, Cantisani V, Gnecchi M, et al. Contrast-enhanced ultrasound examination of the breast: a literature review. Ultraschall Med 2012;33(7):E1–7.

16. Melotti MK, Berg WA. Core needle breast biopsy in patients undergoing anticoagulation therapy: preliminary results. AJR Am J Roentgenol 2000; 174:245–9.

17. Somerville P, Seifert PJ, Destounis SV, et al. Anticoagulation and bleeding risk after core needle biopsy. AJR Am J Roentgenol 2008;191:1194–7.

18. Ciatto S, Cariaggi P, Bulgaresi P. The value of routine cytologic examination of breast cyst fluids. Acta Cytol 1987;31:301–4.

19. Hindle WH, Arias RD, Florentine B, et al. Lack of utility in clinical practice of cytologic examination of nonbloody cyst fluid from palpable breast cysts. Am J Obstet Gynecol 2000;182:1300–5.

20. Smith DN, Kaelin CM, Korbin CD, et al. Impalpable breast cysts: utility of cytologic examination of fluid obtained with radiologically guided aspiration. Radiology 1997;204:149–51.

Ultrasound-Guided Abscess Drainage: Technical and Clinical Aspects

Desi Dennis, MD, Nael Saad, MD*

KEYWORDS

• Ultrasound • Abscess • Drainage

KEY POINTS

- Preparation for percutaneous drainage of a fluid collection requires a thorough review of the patient's clinical history as well as any additional laboratory or radiologic information.
- It is important to select the appropriate transducer to visualize the targeted fluid collection as well as any adjacent structures to avoid, such as bowel loops or vessels.
- Major complications from percutaneous abscess drainage are rare but include pseudoaneurysms, vessel lacerations, and vascular fistulae. Such complications may be avoided with thorough Doppler interrogation of adjacent vasculature before and during the procedure.
- For pelvic collections, transvaginal and transrectal abscess drainage are alternative routes to draining collections bordered by the urinary bladder, reproductive organs, prostate, bowel, or bony structures.

INTRODUCTION

Advancements in ultrasound-guided abscess drainage have benefited patients with a safe and effective minimally invasive alternative to surgical intervention. Ultrasound-guided percutaneous abscess drainage (PAD) has evolved into one of the most widely used methods of patient care provided by interventionalists.[1] PAD technique has been substantially refined since one of the first reported case series of ultrasound-guided percutaneous aspiration of abscesses by Smith and Bartrum in 1974.[2] Five years later, a study published by Gerzof and colleagues[3] using computed tomography (CT) or ultrasound guidance concluded that nonsurgical drainage by percutaneously placed catheters of relatively small size in combination with appropriate antibiotics may suffice for definitive therapy in many abdominal abscesses.

INDICATIONS

Abscess formation results from a variety of causes. Some of the more common causes of abdominal abscess formation include

1. Postoperative complications, including anastomotic biliary leakage
2. Pancreatitis
3. Gangrenous or perforated cholecystitis
4. Diverticulitis or perforated appendicitis
5. Perforated bowel

In 2010, Wallace and colleagues[4] of the Society of Interventional Radiology Standards of Practice Committee concluded that the prerequisites for percutaneous drainage procedures are an abnormal fluid collection and at least one other criterion included in **Box 1**.

Certain clinical and radiographic signs may suggest that a fluid collection is infected. Clinically, patients may present with refractory fevers, persistent abdominal pain, or localized tenderness. Subsequent laboratory workup may reveal leukocytosis or bacteremia. In unstable patients presenting with septic shock, hypotension with tachycardia, decreased urine output, or other signs and symptoms indicating organ dysfunction may manifest. CT has a 96% accuracy for identifying abdominal abscesses.[5] Intravenous contrast is

Section of Vascular and Interventional Radiology, Mallinckrodt Institute of Radiology, Washington University, 510 South Kingshighway Boulevard, St Louis, MO 63110, USA
* Corresponding author.
E-mail address: saadn@mir.wustl.edu

Ultrasound Clin 8 (2013) 117–124
http://dx.doi.org/10.1016/j.cult.2012.12.002
1556-858X/13/$ – see front matter © 2013 Elsevier Inc. All rights reserved.

ultrasound.theclinics.com

routinely given unless contraindicated. Oral contrast for suspected intra-abdominal abscesses can be beneficial, particularly in patients with minimal intraperitoneal fat or to assist diagnosis of a perforated viscus. CT characteristics of an infected fluid collection include wall enhancement (hyperemia) after intravenous contrast and obliteration of adjacent fat planes caused by inflammatory stranding.

Certain instances may require a fluid sample for further characterization. For example, postoperative patients that have undergone a lymph node dissection may subsequently develop a fluid collection. However, the differential diagnosis may include a postoperative lymphocele, seroma, or an abscess. Thus, laboratory analysis of the fluid can guide further therapy, such as catheter placement and alcohol ablation in lymphoceles or antibiotic therapy for infected fluid collections.

A percutaneous catheter may be placed as a temporizing measure before a definitive surgical procedure (**Fig. 1**). This scenario is commonly encountered after postoperative bile leaks,

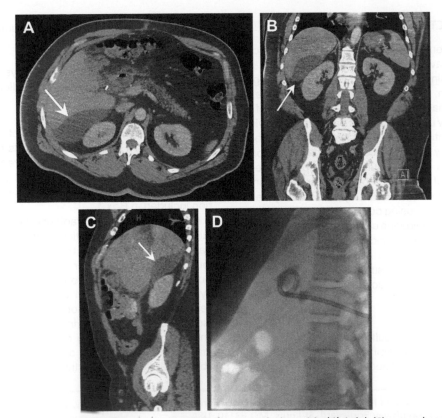

Fig. 1. A 55-year-old man status after cholecystectomy for acute cholecystitis. (*A*) Axial, (*B*) coronal, and (*C*) sagittal contrast-enhance CT images show a partially loculated fluid collection (*arrows*) extending from the gallbladder fossa into the Morrison space. (*D*) Lateral projection fluoroscopic image demonstrates successful placement of a 16F Cope Loop (Cook, Bloomington, Indiana) catheter into the corresponding fluid collection.

including complications from cholecystectomies, liver transplantation, Billroth II procedures, and pancreatic resections.[6] Such iatrogenic bile duct injuries may require reconstruction with a Roux-en-Y hepaticojejunostomy.

There are no absolute contraindications to PAD placement. However, coagulopathy is a relative contraindication that can usually be corrected with the appropriate therapy. A suboptimal window to gain access to a fluid collection, such as a drainage route that traverses pleura or bowel, may also preclude treatment.

There are several advantages of using ultrasound over CT for PAD. Notably, there is no ionizing radiation when such procedures are performed under ultrasound guidance. Although this is beneficial to all patients, alternatives to radiation exposure for children and pregnant patients are especially important. In 2008, Mettler and colleagues[7] reported that the effective dose of an abdominal CT was approximately 8 mSv, which would take 2.7 years to acquire the same effective dose from natural background radiation. Another advantage for selecting ultrasound is the relatively shorter time requirements to complete the procedure. Necessary adjustments while gaining access and subsequent catheter deployment are performed in real time with ultrasound but require frequent rescanning to guarantee accurate placement during CT guidance, thus increasing the total procedure time. Additionally, logistical arrangements are usually simpler with procedures performed under ultrasound guidance. Sonographers are usually not essential to perform the procedure, and ultrasound machines are commonly available when needed. The use of CT scanners often requires reserved time as well as a technologist for operation.

PATIENT PREPARATION

Preparation for percutaneous drainage of a fluid collection requires a thorough review of the patients' clinical history as well as any additional laboratory or radiologic information. If patients are admitted to another service, then consultation with the referring team is necessary to establish a clear indication for the procedure as described earlier. In addition, the patients' coagulation profile should be interrogated. At the authors' institution, the guidelines for nonvascular interventional procedures, including PAD, require an international normalized ratio less than 1.75 and platelets greater than 80 000. The authors discontinue heparin infusions at least 4 hours before the anticipated procedure start time. Furthermore, clopidogrel bisulfate should be discontinued at least 1 week before an elective nonvascular procedure.

Most patients with a suspected abscess usually undergo radiographic imaging before the interventionalist is consulted. A review of all available imaging is instrumental to preprocedural planning. At this time, the optimal approach (preferably the shortest and safest to the fluid collection) as well as patient positioning can be determined.

To obtain consent, the procedure, its alternatives, and potential complications should be discussed with patients. Risks and complications include pain, bleeding, infection, damage to adjacent structures, and allergy to medications. Other risks are included on a case-by-case basis (eg, pneumothorax during a subdiaphragmatic abscess drainage). A preprocedure sedation workup is required on all patients who are likely to receive conscious sedation. The Joint Commission on Accreditation of Healthcare Organizations further mandates that conscious sedation for non–operating room procedures include intraprocedure monitoring and discharge criteria for all patients.[8] Finally, each patient should receive preprocedural broad-spectrum antibiotic coverage to decrease the risk of infectious complications.

ULTRASOUND SETTINGS

It is important to select the right transducer to guide the needle during entry and provide visualization of the targeted fluid collection (**Fig. 2**). In addition, any adjacent structures to avoid, such as bowel loops or vessels, should be adequately visualized. A linear array transducer is advantageous for superficial fluid collections that are located within 5 cm of the skin surface given its superior resolution. For smaller acoustic windows or drainages requiring an intercostal approach, a phased array transducer may be necessary because of its smaller size. Curved array transducers are often used given its ability for better penetration and deeper imaging. Properly selected machine settings are also important to optimally visualize deep fluid collections. In 2009, a study by Petar Avramovski[9] demonstrated that unadjusted focus and time gain control led to more cases of missed deep liver level abscesses. The focal zone is the point at which the ultrasound beam is at its narrowest and represents the point of greatest intensity and best lateral resolution. The time gain compensation corrects for increased attenuation of sound with tissue depth.

CATHETER SELECTION

The size, location, and viscosity of the fluid collection are several factors that dictate catheter selection. In addition, kink resistance, securing mechanism, tip design, and cost are other features

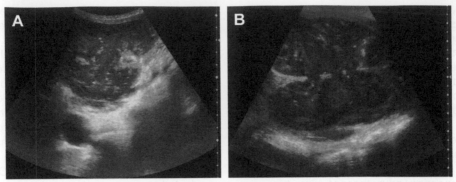

Fig. 2. A 51-year-old man with a right upper quadrant abdominal abscess. (*A*) Longitudinal gray-scale sonographic image of the right upper quadrant with a curved array transducer demonstrates an irregular hypoechoic collection with internal debris. (*B*) A similar image obtained with a linear array transducer after adjusting the focal zone better delineates the margins and demonstrates the bilobed nature of the abscess.

taken into consideration before ultimately choosing a catheter. At the authors' institution, Multipurpose Cope Loop and Dawson-Mueller catheters (Cook, Bloomington, Indiana) are frequently used given their easy-to-use locking mechanism and large, oval side ports to facilitate drainage capability (**Fig. 3**).

Dawson-Mueller catheters are used for smaller fluid collections because of their smaller loop diameter (10 mm) compared with the larger Multipurpose Cope Loop pigtail diameter of 25 mm.

Both catheters can be deployed using the Seldinger technique or one-stick trocar introduction system. The authors commonly use Thal drainage catheters (Cook, Bloomington, Indiana) for larger abscesses and collections containing viscous or debris-laden fluid. Thal catheters have several large, oval side ports and are available up to 24F to facilitate drainage. Sump dual-lumen catheters contain a second lumen that allows air to pass to the distal tip of the catheter, theoretically reducing negative pressure and improving the free flow of

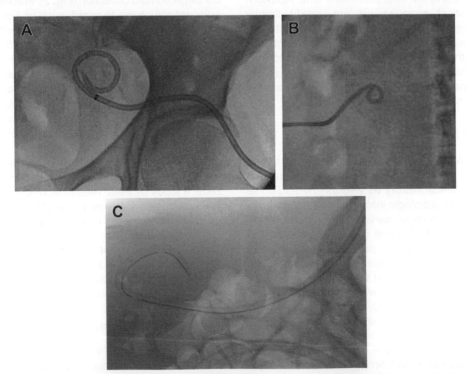

Fig. 3. Fluoroscopic images of the (*A*) Cope Loop, (*B*) Dawson Mueller, and (*C*) Thal catheters (Cook, Bloomington, Indiana).

fluid. However, a study by Hoyt and colleagues[10] evaluating the efficiency of double-lumen sump catheters and single-lumen catheters in vitro concluded that single-lumen catheters performed as well as or more efficiently than double-lumen sump catheters of the same outer diameter.

TECHNIQUE

After using maximum sterile barriers, prepping the skin overlying the fluid collection, and interrogation of the abscess with ultrasound, gaining access to the targeted collection is the next step. Generally, 2 widely used techniques are used, the Seldinger technique and use of a one-stick trocar introduction system. With the Seldinger technique, a sharp hollow needle, preferably 18-gauge or larger, is inserted into the targeted collection under ultrasound guidance. Placing the needle immediately next to the side of the transducer will position the needle in the plane of the image and allow visualization of the needle shaft and tip during entry (**Fig. 4**). Attaching a syringe to the needle may verify successful access if aspiration yields fluid.

Additionally, injecting a small amount of dilute contrast under fluoroscopy can confirm the location by opacifying the cavity. Once the needle is in place, a guidewire is advanced through the needle and coiled in the collection to maintain purchase while the needle is removed. The tract is then dilated to accommodate the diameter of the selected catheter. Subsequently, the catheter is advanced over the guidewire, formed in the collection (if necessary), then secured in place (**Fig. 5**). A one-stick trocar introduction system consists of a catheter mounted on a solid needle (trocar), which is inserted into the fluid collection as one unit. Visualization of the guiding needle during placement is imperative because redirecting the catheter-trocar unit generates more localized trauma when compared with needle redirection during the Seldinger technique. Once the catheter-trocar unit is accurately placed in the targeted collection, the catheter is deployed into the collection and the trocar is removed. An obvious disadvantage of the trocar technique is the difficulty repositioning the drainage catheter once deployed. The trocar technique is feasible for small- and intermediate-sized catheters; however, larger catheters (greater than 16F) are not equipped with a trocar needle.

COMPLICATIONS

Major complications from PAD are rare. Transient bacteremia resulting from the spillage of infected contents into the bloodstream is seen in up to 5% of cases.[11] As stated previously, preprocedural broad-spectrum antibiotic coverage is essential; subsequent antibiotics should be selected by the cultures taken from the abscess cavity. Another complication involves bleeding while initially gaining access into the fluid collection or after catheter placement.

Pseudoaneurysms, vessel lacerations, and vascular fistulae are complications that may require additional treatment, such as transcatheter embolization to control bleeding. Such complications may be avoided with thorough Doppler interrogation of adjacent vasculature before and during the procedure. Severe peritonitis is a major complication that could result from unintentional catheterization through the colon and can progress to septic shock. If transcolonic catheterization leads to only minor clinical sequela, then the catheter may remain in place until a mature tract has developed.

Differentiating the bowel signature from adjacent structures on ultrasound and reviewing pertinent anatomy on preprocedural cross-sectional imaging can reduce inadvertent catheter placement caused by operator error. Normal bowel signature has a 3-layer pattern that is usually

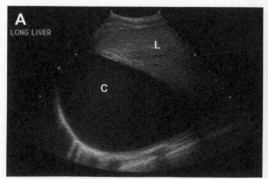
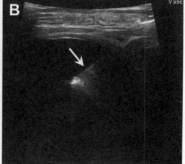

Fig. 4. A 6-year-old boy with a hepatic subcapsular fluid collection after lacerating liver from a bicycle injury. (*A*) Longitudinal gray-scale ultrasound image shows a large hepatic subcapsular collection (C) with mass effect on the liver parenchyma (L). (*B*) Ultrasound-guided needle access with visualization of the needle shaft and tip (*arrow*).

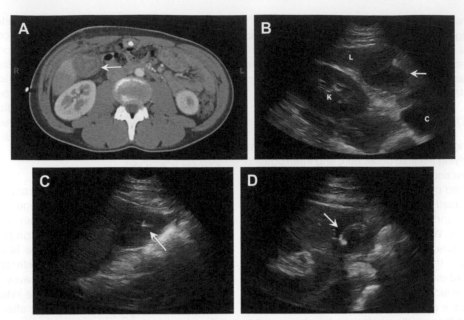

Fig. 5. A 23-year-old man with a subhepatic abscess following a bile duct iatrogenic injury during cholecystectomy. (A) Transaxial contrast-enhanced CT image demonstrates a fluid collection (arrow) anterior to the right kidney between the liver and colon. (B) Axial gray-scale ultrasound image of the fluid collection (arrow) flanked by the liver, right kidney, and colon. Subsequent gray-scale axial ultrasound images showing (C) needle access (arrow) and (D) placement of a pigtail drainage catheter (arrow). C, colon; K, right kidney; L, liver.

recognizable by ultrasound.[12] The innermost distinct echogenic rind is comprised of mucosa and submucosa surrounding the bowel lumen. The muscularis propria produces a hypoechoic layer. The outermost adventitia/serosa and adjacent fat produces an outer echogenic layer (Fig. 6).

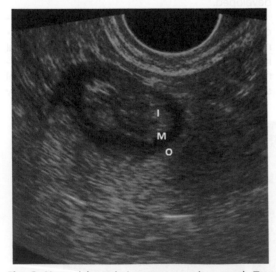

Fig. 6. Normal bowel signature on ultrasound. Two echogenic layers are separated by a hypoechoic muscular layer. I, inner mucosa and submucosa layer; M, middle muscularis layer; O, outer adventitia/serosa/surrounding fat layer.

PELVIC FLUID COLLECTIONS

Visceral structures in the deep pelvis may complicate a transabdominal approach to a fluid collection. Transvaginal (TVAD) and transrectal abscess drainage (TRAD) (Fig. 7) are alternative routes to draining collections bordered by the urinary bladder, reproductive organs, prostate, bowel, or bony structures. TRADs and TVADs are placed with an endoluminal transducer under ultrasound guidance. At the authors' institution, they routinely use an 18-gauge Ring needle (Cook, Bloomington, Indiana) to access the fluid collection and then use the Seldinger or trocar technique for catheter placement. Patients may be somewhat apprehensive about having a TRAD or TVAD placed; however, the catheter is usually well tolerated.[13] An obvious disadvantage of using an endocavitary route is the inability to perform the procedure sterilely, risking contamination from natural flora while gaining access or during catheter placement.

A transgluteal approach is another commonly used route for pelvic abscess drainage. This route may be preferable if there is clinical suspicion that the pelvic collection may be sterile. There is some disagreement in the literature concerning the severity and persistence of pain while placing a transgluteal catheter compared with an endocavitary route.[14] The catheter should pass medially and inferiorly within the greater sciatic foramen to

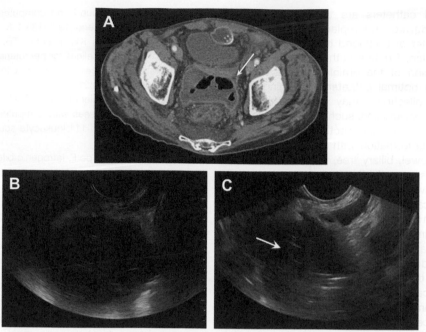

Fig. 7. A 65-year-old man status after total colectomy and ileorectal anastomosis complicated by a pelvic abscess. (*A*) Transaxial contrast-enhanced CT image reveals a collection of fluid and gas anterior to the rectum and posterior to the urinary bladder (*arrow*). (*B*) Gray-scale ultrasound image corresponding to the fluid collection on CT. (*C*) Gray-scale ultrasound image demonstrating transrectal needle access (*arrow*) of the fluid collection with subsequent catheter placement.

decrease the incidence of going through the piriformis muscle or sacral plexus, which have been shown to increase the incidence of pelvic and leg pain.[15]

POSTPROCEDURAL CARE AND MANAGEMENT

It is important to obtain fluoroscopic images after catheter insertion to document the placement and acquire baseline imaging for patients who will require subsequent follow-up. Once the catheter is in place, it can either be connected to bulb suction or a bag for gravity drainage. The interventionalist should aspirate as much fluid as possible during the initial catheter placement. Patients are instructed to flush the catheter daily with normal saline to maintain a patent lumen for drainage. This practice is particularly important when draining viscous or debris-filled collections, such as pancreatic abscesses containing necrotic material. However, flushing the catheter is contraindicated when there is suspicion of a fistulous connection. In this scenario, flushing will keep the fistulous communication open and delay healing.

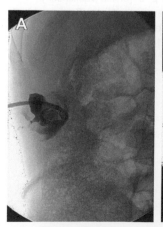
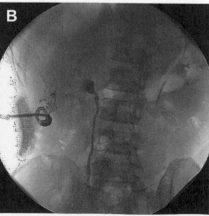

Fig. 8. A 51-year-old man with a right upper quadrant abdominal abscess whose ultrasound images were demonstrated earlier (see Fig. 2). (*A*) Initial placement of a 12F Mac Lock pigtail catheter into a moderate-sized right upper quadrant abscess cavity. (*B*) There is near complete resolution of the abscess cavity 13 days later. The drainage catheter was subsequently removed.

Occluded catheters are typically exchanged over a guidewire and replaced with a similar-sized catheter or upgraded to facilitate drainage and resolution. Routine catheter checks assess the regression of the draining abscess pocket and ensure optimal catheter positioning. Some complex collections may require additional cross-sectional imaging, such as CT, to document the evolution. Contrast injection aids the evaluation of fistula formation with adjacent structures, including bowel, biliary tree, or vasculature. This evaluation is essential if daily output substantially increases over a period of time.

The clinical course dictates when the drainage catheter can be removed. Patients should be afebrile and show improvement in leukocytosis if initially present. Drainage from the cavity should be less than 10 mL daily from a patent catheter. Additionally, injection of the catheter must demonstrate resolution of the cavity. If these criteria are met, then the catheter can be removed and a sterile dressing can be placed over the entry site (**Fig. 8**). Minimal drainage from the catheter tract is allowed during the first 24 hours; however, persistent drainage for several days may require further evaluation.

SUMMARY

Ultrasound-guided PAD is a safe and effective alternative to surgical intervention. A general understanding of the necessary patient preparation, ultrasound optimization, catheter insertion techniques, and postprocedural care can limit potential complications and lead to successful minimally invasive treatment of abscesses.

REFERENCES

1. vanSonnenberg E, Wittich GR, Goodacre BW, et al. Percutaneous abscess drainage: an update. World J Surg 2001;25:362–72.
2. Smith EH, Bartrum RJ Jr. Ultrasonically guided percutaneous aspiration of abscesses. AJR Am J Roentgenol 1974;122:308–12.
3. Gerzof SG, Robbins AH, Birkett DH, et al. Percutaneous catheter drainage of abdominal abscesses guided by ultrasound and computed tomography. AJR Am J Roentgenol 1979;133:1–8.
4. Wallace MJ, Chin KW, Fletcher TB, et al. Quality improvement guidelines for percutaneous drainage/aspiration of abscess and fluid collections. J Vasc Interv Radiol 2010;21:431–5.
5. Knochel JQ, Koehler PR, Lee TG, et al. Diagnosis of abdominal abscesses with computed tomography, ultrasound, and in-111 leukocyte scans. Radiology 1980;137:425–32.
6. Jablonska B, Lampe P. Iatrogenic bile duct injuries: etiology, diagnosis, and management. World J Gastroenterol 2009;15(33):4097–104.
7. Mettler FA Jr, Huda W, Yoshizumi TT, et al. Effective doses in radiology and diagnostic nuclear medicine: a catalog. Radiology 2008;248(1):254–63.
8. Procedure for intravenous conscious sedation. Comprehensive accreditation manual for hospitals: the official handbook. Oakbrook Terrace (IL): The Joint Commission on Accreditation of Healthcare Organizations; 1999.
9. Avramovski P. Value of ultrasound machine settings optimization for better diagnosis of focal liver lesions. Maced J Med Sci 2009;2(2):149–52.
10. Hoyt AC, D'Agostino HB, Carrillo AJ, et al. Drainage efficiency of double-lumen sump catheters and single-lumen catheters: an in-vitro comparison. J Vasc Interv Radiol 1997;8(2):267–70.
11. Lorenz J, Thomas JL. Complications of percutaneous fluid drainage. Semin Intervent Radiol 2006; 23(2):194–204.
12. Brant WE. The core curriculum: ultrasound. Philadelphia: Lippincott Williams & Wilkins; 2001.
13. Hovsepian DM, Steele JR, Malden ES. Transrectal verses transvaginal abscess drainage: survey of patient tolerance and effect on activities of daily living. Radiology 1999;212(1):159–63.
14. Lorenz JM, Ray CE Jr, Burke CT, et al. Expert panel on interventional radiology. ACR Appropriateness Criteria® radiologic management of infected fluid collections. Reston (VA): American College of Radiology (ACR); 2011. p. 8. [online publication].
15. Walser E, Raza S, Hernandez A, et al. Sonographically guided transgluteal drainage of pelvic abscesses. Am J Roentgenol 2003;181:498–500.

Dysfunctional Transjugular Intrahepatic Portosystemic Shunt

Anatomic Defects and Doppler Ultrasound Evaluation

William P. Brehmer, MD, Wael E. Saad, MD, FSIR*

KEYWORDS

- Transjugular intrahepatic portosystemic shunt (TIPS) • Doppler studies • Portal hypertension
- Covered stent (PTFE)

KEY POINTS

- Doppler ultrasound provides limited visualization of in-stent stenoses in TIPS created by covered-stents in the first 24 to 48 hours after TIPS creation. However, proof of mere patency can be made by proving portal vein patency and and flow direction and TIPS hepatic venous outflow.
- Intra-stent (in-stent) stenosis has become a less common finding in the covered-stent era of TIPS creation.
- Most stenoses in the covered stent era can be avoided with good TIPS creation technique and operator experience.
- Hepatic venous outflow stenoses have become the main site of TIPS stenoses in the covered stent era of TIPS creation.
- The same Doppler parameters for evaluating TIPS created by bare-stents apply to TIPS created by covered stents.

BACKGROUND AND INTRODUCTION

Liver disease and managing the complications of cirrhotic patients is often challenging. The majority of these complications are a result of portal hypertension. Since the introduction of the expandable stent, the creation of TIPS has become a widely accepted treatment of the complications of portal hypertension. Indications for tips creation include intractable ascites, hepatic hydrothorax, hemorrhage from gastroesophageal varices, hepatorenal syndrome, and Budd-Chiari syndrome.[1,2] Often, intractable ascites and variceal bleeding that have failed medical management or less-invasive management (repeat paracentesis and endoscopic

hemostatic measures, respectively) are the most common reasons for TIPS placement.

Not everyone is a candidate for TIPS placement. Contraindications include severe hepatic encephalopathy due to the potential for worsening encephalopathy. Other contraindications include severe right heart failure due to the possibility of exasperating a patient's symptoms. Relative contraindications include chronic thrombosis or cavernous transformation of the portal vein due to potential technical challenges. In addition, active systemic or hepatic infections and hypervascular liver tumors are considered relative contraindications.[3,4] Moreover, poor hepatic reserve (reduced

Division of Vascular Interventional Radiology, Department of Imaging Sciences, University of Virginia Health System, PO Box 800170, Charlottesville, VA 22908, USA
* Corresponding author.
E-mail address: WS6R@virginia.edu

Ultrasound Clin 8 (2013) 125–135
http://dx.doi.org/10.1016/j.cult.2012.12.004
1556-858X/13/$ – see front matter © 2013 Elsevier Inc. All rights reserved.

synthetic function) can also be a contraindication for elective TIPS creation.

Lowering the portosystemic gradient to a level less than 12 mm Hg is the widely accepted desired intraprocedural endpoint with technical and hemodynamic (gradient <12 mm Hg) success rates reported greater than 90%.[5–8] Improved control of ascites and control of bleeding varices occur in up to 80% to 90% of patients after TIPS placement.[3–5,9,10] Maintaining stent patency is critical, however, in preventing the return of symptoms or developing other complications related to portal hypertension. This was particularly true for bare stents that were placed in the first decade of TIPS practice (1993–2003). The original bare-metal stents that were used for TIPS creation had poor patency rates of approximately 40% to 60% at 1 year.[10,11] Since the introduction of the expanded polytetrafluoroethylene (e-PTFE)–covered stent, primary patency rates have significantly improved to a reported approximately 80% to 84% at 1 year.[12] Today, with the advent of commercially available covered stents specifically designed for TIPS (Viatorr stent, W. L. Gore & Associates, Flagstaff, Arizona), the PTFE-covered stent is used almost exclusively when creating TIPS and is the focus of this article.

If a hemodynamic abnormality is suspected clinically or by noninvasive imaging, then the shunt can be evaluated with the gold standard, portal venography. Portal venography allows visualization of the stent, ability to measure pressure gradients across the stent, and potentially revising the shunt if necessary. Unfortunately, venography is invasive and expensive, which argues for an effective screening protocol to prevent unnecessary invasive testing. Moreover, preventing the complications of TIPS malfunction rather than managing the clinical consequences after malfunction is paramount. For this reason, an appropriate screening modality that is noninvasive, inexpensive, and readily available is necessary. In addition, screening is important because stent revision is often technically successful. Doppler ultrasound has proved an effective screening modality.[13–16] With the advent of the improved patency covered stent, however, there has not been a clear consensus on standardization of when Doppler ultrasound screening should be performed.[13–16]

TIPS ANATOMY AND DEFINITIONS

The new Viatorr covered stent used to create a TIPS is a metallic partially covered stent that is placed bridging the portal venous circulation and the hepatic venous outflow (hepatic vein) (Fig. 1A). The TIPS is vertically oriented (along the long axis

of the human body), parallel, straight, or curved, to the vertebral column. When curved, its convexity is usually toward the posterolateral (posterior and/or lateral) aspect of the patient (see Fig. 1A). Where and at what angle in the portal vein the stent enters (the TIPS landing) and where the TIPS exits the hepatic venous outflow determine its configuration and course. This varies considerably from one operator to another and from one TIPS to another with the same operator. Moreover, the portal venous entry can be in the left portal vein or the right portal vein, and this determines expected reversals of flow, if any, in the ipsilateral portal vein (discussed later). As a result, in the authors' opinion, it is important for sonographers and diagnostic radiologists to look at the completion portal venograms to understand the shape, configuration, and laterality of the TIPS they evaluate by Doppler ultrasound.

In addition, it is not uncommon for radiologists evaluating TIPS to refer to the TIPS ends as *proximal and distal ends*. This can create confusion when referring to ends that are stenotic on ultrasound. This is because some radiologists may refer to the portal venous end (PVE) as proximal (proximal to flow) or distal (distal relative to a patient's body).[17] Similarly, radiologists referr to the hepatic venous end (HVE) as distal (distal to flow) or proximal (proximal relative to the patient's body). Strictly speaking, when referring to a vessel or conduit with flow within it (as in the case of TIPS), proximal and distal always are in reference to normal (expected) blood flow. Nevertheless, to prevent confusion, the authors recommend referring to the TIPS ends as PVE and HVE (see Fig. 1B, C).[17] The term, *hepatic venous outflow*, refers to the HVE of the stent, the unstented hepatic vein (if any) distal to the HVE with or without the inferior vena cava (see Fig. 1D).

ANATOMIC DEFECTS OF TIPS IN THE COVERED STENT ERA

Anatomic defects associated with TIPS refers to narrowings of any sort (ingrowth stenoses and/or structural kinks) and occlusions (and their sites) that are associated with TIPS. It is important for diagnostic radiologists and sonographers to understand these issues. The incidence of occurrence of anatomic defects in TIPS has been reduced considerably with the use of covered stents.[17] Moreover, the prevalence of particular locations has changed with the advent of covered stents.[17] Before the use of covered stents, bare stents were permeable to bile that seeped from microbiliary to TIPS fistulae, which accelerated pseudointimal hyperplasia.[17] In addition, bile is thrombogenic and may lead to TIPS thrombosis.

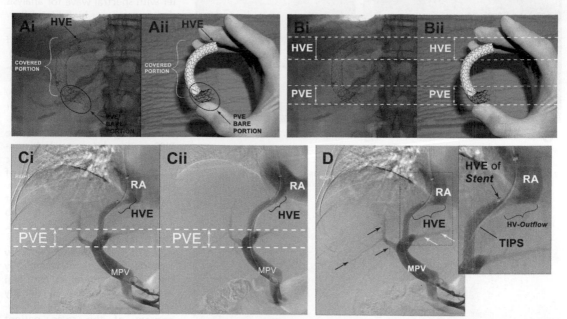

Fig. 1. TIPS stent anatomy and definitions. (*A*). The shunt is composed of at least 1 stent. The Viatorr stent is the most commonly used covered stent graft (covered stent) and is the only TIPS-approved commercially available stent. It is composed of a self-expanding chain-link (flexible) bare portion, which is placed in the portal venous system. This bare portion (always 2 cm in length) is self-expanding and is constrained by an outer sheath only and thus is released by unsheathing. The covered portion is covered with e-PTFE on the inside of a frame, which is formed of a spiraling ring of nitinol. The covered portion varies in length and is also self-expanding. It is constrained, however, by a suture line and is deployed by pulling on the cord connected to the suture line. The tip (relative to the TIPS) of the covered stent is referred to as the HVE of the TIPS. (*B*) The shunt bridges the portal venous system and the hepatic venous system and is vertically oriented relative to the long axis of the human body. The end of the shunt at the portal vein is referred to as the PVE and the end at the hepatic venous outflow vein is called the HVE. The shunt (TIPS) can be curved or straight and varies considerably in curvature and course. If it curves, it usually curves with its convexity toward the posterolateral aspect. (*C*) Two digitally subtracted portal venograms in sequence demonstrate the PVE on the side of the MPV and the HVE, which ultimately empties into the right atrium (RA). (*D*) This is a TIPS bridging between the left portal vein and the right hepatic vein. The HVE of the stent falls short of the hepatocaval junction. The unstented hepatic vein is labeled the HV-Outflow, which also comprises the RA. Notice the right portal venous branches/radicals (*black arrows*) and the left portal venous branches/radicals (*white arrows*) after TIPS creation. Opacifying these branches varies considerably based on the site of the TIPS, how wide the TIPS is dilated, the liver resistance, and how powerful the contrast injection is.

Stenoses in TIPS created by bare stents have occurred throughout the course of the TIPS as well as the hepatic venous outflow.[17,18] There are 2 reasons why TIPS patency has improved since approximately 2003. First is the use of covered stents (discussed later) and second is the understanding that extending the TIPS stent (bare stent or covered stent) to the hepatocaval junction (within 1 cm from it is acceptable) reduces the incidence of hepatic venous outflow stenosis.[17,18] Covered stents that are covered with e-PTFE prevent the seepage of bile from microbiliary fistuale and have considerably reduced stenoses along the parenchymal tract (central portion) of the TIPS.[17] The reduction of proximal and central (parencymal tract) stenoses, however, has increased the prevalence of HVE (hepatic venous outflow distal to the distal end of the stent)

(**Fig. 2**).[17] Proximal stenoses at the PVE of the TIPS still can occur with covered stents if the Viatorr stent is pulled excessively where the bare portion is dragged into the proximal parenchymal tract, which no longer becomes covered by e-PTFE (**Fig. 3**).[17] As can be deduced, both HVE and PVE stenoses can be prevented with good technique (not pulling the stent excessively and making sure that the TIPS is extended to within 1 cm from the hepatocaval junction).[17,18] Covered stents have not completely prevented intrastent/parenchymal tract stenoses but they have reduced these lesions considerably, which are referred to as diffuse narrowing (stenoses) (**Fig. 4**).[17] The exact cause and pathology of these intrastent stenoses is unknown. It can only be speculated as to the pathology and etiology of these stenoses. The cause may be (1) due to faulty

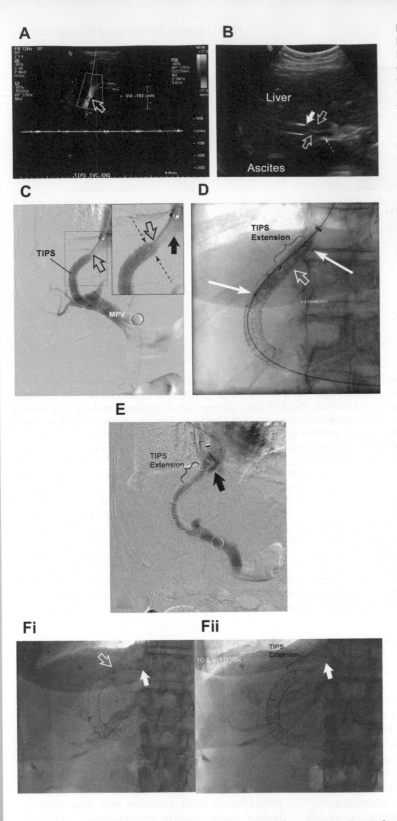

Fig. 2. HVE stenosis: gray-scale and Doppler findings. (*A*) Color Doppler with spectral wave for analysis demonstrating a high blood flow velocity of 192 cm/s (normal: 80–90 to 180–190 cm/s) at the HVE of the TIPS (*hollow white arrow*). This has increased from prior examination by 60 cm/s (prior examination velocity was approximately 130 cm/s). This is suspicious for HVE stenosis. (*B*) Gray-scale ultrasound image at the HVE of the TIPS (*solid white arrow*) demonstrating a bare (unstented) hepatic vein (*dashed arrow*) and an area of narrowing (*between hollow arrows*) just distal to the HVE of the stent (*solid white arrow*). Also noticed was new-onset ascites. These are all collaborative evidence of a hepatic venous outflow stenosis that is hemodynamically significant (see parameters of [*A*]) as well as potentially functionally significant (*ascites*). (*C*) Portal venogram of the same patient demonstrated that the HVE of the TIPS stent (*between dashed arrows*) falls short of the hepatocaval junction (*solid black arrow*) and there is a narrowing in the hepatic venous outflow (*hollow arrows*) as predicted by the ultrasound examination. It is believed that hepatic venous outflow narrowings by uncovered (unstented) hepatic veins is due to neointimal hyperplasia of the hepatic venous lining in response to high velocity and turbid flow in the outflow hepatic veins. The hepatic veins respond by this because they are not designed for high and turbid flow. This is along the lines of hepatic venous outflow stenoses in dialysis conduits. (*D*) The HVE of the TIPS was extended (TIPS extension) with another Viatorr stent to the hepatocaval junction. The stent covered the site of the hepatic venous outflow narrowing (*hollow arrow*) and was ballooned with an 8-mm balloon (*between solid white arrows*). The portosystemic gradient dropped from 15 mm Hg (24 mm Hg in portal vein and 9 mm Hg in the right atrium) to 4 mm Hg (11 mm Hg in portal vein and 7 mm Hg in the right atrium). (*E*) Post-TIPS revision digitally subtracted portal venogram using carbon dioxide as a contrast agent demonstrates resolution of the hepatic venous outflow narrowing with by the new TIPS stent extension. The new tips HVE falls (lands) closer (within 1 cm) to the hepatocaval junction (*solid black arrow*). (*F*) Two spot fluoroscopic images before (*Fi*) and after (*Fii*) the TIPS revision with the additional TIPS extension. The images demonstrate the details of the stents. The original HVE (*Fi: hollow arrow*) was a distance (>2 cm) from the hepatocaval junction (*Fi: solid white arrow*) and after the extension it is near the hepatocaval junction (*Fii: solid white arrow*).

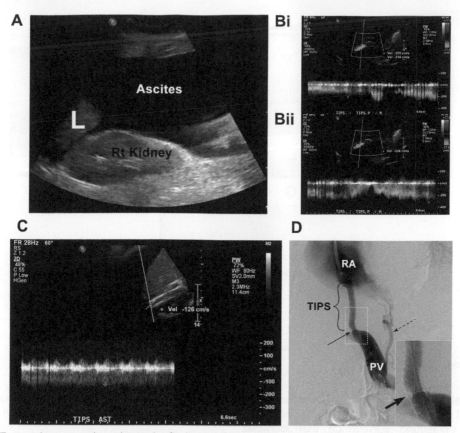

Fig. 3. PVE stenosis: gray-scale and Doppler findings. (*A*) Gray-scale ultrasound image demonstrating moderate to significant new onset ascites after 16 months from the original TIPS creation. L, liver; Rt Kidney, right kidney. (*B*) Color Doppler with spectral wave for analysis demonstrating blood flow velocity of 205 cm/s to 324 cm/s (normal: 80–90 to 180–190 cm/s) at the PVE of the TIPS. This is suspicious for a PVE stenosis. (*C*) Color Doppler with spectral wave for analysis demonstrating a high blood flow velocity of 126 cm/s (normal: 80–90 to 180–190 cm/s) distally within the stent of the TIPS (mid to distal or mid to HVE). This is a blood flow reduction within the TIPS of at least 75 cm/s. This is collaborative evidence of a significant stenosis at the PVE of the TIPS. (*D*) Portal venogram of the same patient demonstrated that the PVE of the TIPS stent (*solid black arrow*) has a narrowing as predicted by the ultrasound examination. At this projection, the stenosis appears to be right at the portal venous entry site. Another sign that the stenosis is of hemodynamic significance is the appearance of filling of the left gastric vein (*dashed black arrow*). PV, main portal vein; RA, right atrium. (*E*) Magnified and obliqued portal venogram of the same patient so as to profile the portal entry site of the Viatorr stent. The image demonstrated that the junction (radio-opaque ring) between the bare portion and covered portion of the Viatorr stent is pulled back from the portal venous entry site. There is pseudointimal hyperplasia (*hollow arrows*) causing narrowing at the PVE of the TIPS. The portosystemic gradient was 21 mm Hg (26 mm Hg in portal vein and 5 mm Hg in the right atrium). (*F*) Two spot fluoroscopic images during (*Fi*) and after (*Fii*) the TIPS revision with the additional portal venous covered stent TIPS extension. The e-PTFE coverage is marked by the annotated brackets and now the e-PTFE coverage is extended across the portal venous entry site. The portosystemic gradient dropped from 21 mm Hg (26 mm Hg in portal vein and 5 mm Hg in the right atrium) to 4 mm Hg (16 mm Hg in portal vein and 12 mm Hg in the right atrium). (*G*) Magnified and obliqued portal venogram of the same patient so as to profile the portal entry site of the Viatorr stent extension is shown. The image demonstrated extension of the new Viatorr stent, with its e-PTFE covering across the portal venous entry site and resolution of the PVE stenosis (*hollow arrow*).

e-PTFE that becomes porous and allows biliary leaks and tissue in-growth; (2) propagation of neo-intimal and/or pseudointimal hyperplasia from the ends (hepatic end or, most likely, portal end); or (3) diffuse laminar thrombosis without tissue in-growth. The other cause of TIPS dysfunction is TIPS thrombosis. Anecdotally, this has probably

not changed in incidence since the switching of TIPS creation from bare stents to covered stents. The causes of TIPS thrombosis include (1) hemo-dynamic phenomenon, such as competing shunts, leading to stasis of flow and subsequent throm-bosis; (2) hypercoagulable states; and (3) ne-glected significant stenoses that lead to blood

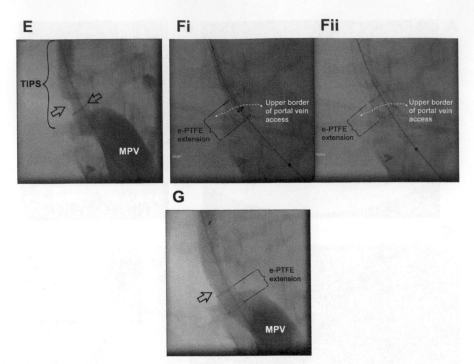

Fig. 3. (*continued*)

flow stasis and thrombosis. The latter (TIPS stenoses) should be prevented by adequate Doppler ultrasound surveillance that identifies stenoses before they become critical to blood flow.

DOPPLER ULTRASOUND SURVEILLANCE
Timing of Surveillance

In the covered stent era of TIPS creation, there is no clear consensus as to at what intervals after TIPS creation Doppler ultrasound examinations should be performed. If a patient has new or recurrent symptoms related to portal hypertension, an ultrasound may reveal a possible explanation. Routine screening of asymptomatic patients varies, however, from institution to institution. An institution with a large experience with TIPS screening suggests routine screening 24 to 48 hours postplacement; then at 3, 6, and 12 months; and then annually thereafter.[19] Ultrasound within the first few days after TIPS placement can be difficult due to the gas associated with the covered stent and the artifacts created by the gas. The gas (air) is initially entrapped in the e-PTFE during manufacturing and it takes 24 to 72 hours (sometimes more) for air bubbles to resolve and be replaced by bodily fluid/tissue (referred to as *gas denucleation*). For this reason, waiting a couple days to perform the initial ultrasound is a reasonable practice. Institutions that perform a 24-hours to 48-hours Doppler ultrasound post-TIPS

consider this examination a baseline examination for subsequent examination comparison.

Portohepatic Hemodynamics

Familiarity with a few of the important hemodynamic changes that occur after TIPS placement is important. The shunt provides a way for the existing high-pressure portal system to bypass the liver and flow into the lower-pressure systemic venous system. Theoretically, this flow diversion should allow blood flow in the right and left portal veins to flow towards the stent and away from the liver (hepatofugal flow). Due to the decrease in liver resistance, flow increases within the main portal vein (MPV). The direction of the MPV flow should be toward the liver, that is, hepatopetal.[20,21] Within the liver, the portal venous blood is no longer delivering oxygen to the parenchyma. As a result, the arterial flow increases to maintain adequate oxygenation.[22] This causes increased flow in the hepatic artery.

Gray-scale Ultrasound

Careful gray-scale and color Doppler ultrasound evaluation of the stent morphology and the position relative to prior imaging may be the simplest way to detect an abnormal shunt. If adequately imaged, simple gray-scale and color flow potentially can detect a kink, narrowed lumen (see **Fig. 2**B), abnormal color aliasing, or potential

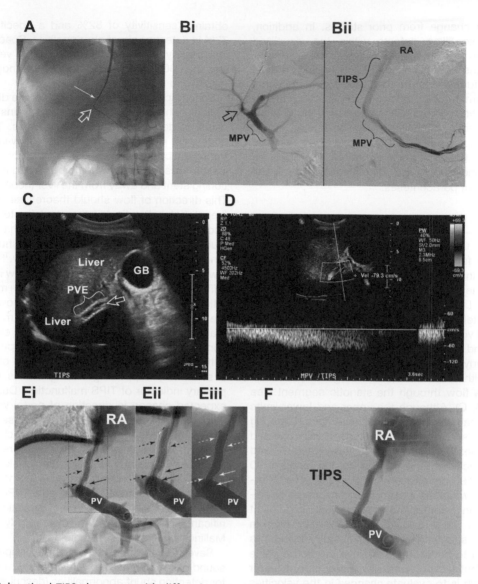

Fig. 4. Suboptimal TIPS placement with diffuse intrastent stenosis: gray-scale and Doppler findings. (*A*) Fluoroscopic spot image during TIPS creation demonstrating that the portal entry is angulated (*hollow arrow*). The wire delineates this as it is passed through the Colapinto needle (*arrow*). (*B*) Portal venogram of the same patient before (*Bi*) and after (*Bii*) the Viatorr stent placement. The images again demonstrated the angulation at the portal venous entry site (*Bi: hollow arrow*). In addition, the TIPS is actually in a portal venous branch (*Bii*). When the TIPS is placed in portal branches (especially in portal branches that are less than 8-mm in diameter), the portal branches can have a significant constricting effect on the TIPS. This constricting effect is even more significant than the constricting effect of the transhepatic parenchymal tract. In other words, it is easier to force dilate the stent within the parenchymal tract than it is along the long axis of a portal venous branch. (*C*) Gray-scale ultrasound image demonstrating intrastent filling defect (*hollow arrow*) after 24 months from the original TIPS creation. The filling defect is near the PVE of the TIPS. (*D*) Color Doppler with spectral wave for analysis demonstrating blood flow velocity of 79 cm/s (normal: 80–90 to 180–190 cm/s) in the midportion of the TIPS. This is a reduction of 70 cm/s from a prior Doppler ultrasound examination and is suspicious for a PVE stenosis. (*E*) Portal venogram of the same patient demonstrated a diffuse narrowing along the entire TIPS. The narrowing is most significant at the PVE of the TIPS stent (*solid arrows*). There is narrowing, however, in the mid to distal TIPS (*dashed arrows*). The portosystemic gradient was 13 mm Hg (18 mm Hg in portal vein and 5 mm Hg in the right atrium). (*F*) Digitally subtracted portogram of the TIPS after TIPS revision with balloon angioplasty demonstrating TIPS patency and resolution of the previously noted diffuse narrowing of the TIPS. The portosystemic gradient dropped from 13 mm Hg (18 mm Hg in portal vein and 5 mm Hg in the right atrium) to 7 mm Hg (18 mm Hg in portal vein and 11 mm Hg in the right atrium). GB, gallbladder; PV, main portal vein; RA, right atrium.

position change from prior studies. In addition, echogenic filling defects within the visualized TIPS can represent significant stenosis or thrombosis (see **Fig. 4**C). Any of these findings should lead to further interrogation with Doppler spectral waveform tracings and possibly guiding further diagnostic work-up. Similarly, a gray-scale ultrasound finding of new or worsening ascites should raise suspicion of possible shunt malfunction (see **Fig. 2**B; **Fig. 3**A). Lack of ascites on grey-scale ultrasound should be clinically correlated with any recent paracenteses.

Doppler Ultrasound Parameters

Several ultrasound parameters have been described for evaluating TIPS. Some of the more useful and accepted parameters are discussed later. The accepted assessment requires the use of color Doppler ultrasound to measure velocities and determine the direction of flow. Measuring in-stent velocities has been one of the most widely used and studied parameters. The concept is that a hemodynamically significant stenosis decreases flow within the nonstenotic segments and increases flow through the stenotic segment (see **Fig. 3**B, C). Although the upper and lower limits of normal stent velocities have varied among different studies, in a large study, Kanterman and colleagues[16] obtained a sensitivity of 82% and a specificity of 72% using a normal range of 90 cm/s o 190 cm/s (see **Figs. 3** and **4**). The difference between the maximum and minimum velocities within a stent is known as the velocity gradient and this value should be abnormally high in stenotic shunts. This particular study found this criterion to have a high positive predictive value (82%) but lacked sensitivity.[16] Perhaps a better approach is to evaluate changes in the velocities over time. Dodd and colleagues[23] showed that using an increase or decrease of 50 cm/s has a good sensitivity of 93% and a specificity of 77% (see **Fig. 2**A; **Fig. 4**D). Other groups have had similar results using slightly different velocities.[16] Monitoring velocity changes makes obtaining an accurate baseline minimal and maximal velocity important.

A temporal change in velocity within the MPV has also received attention for possible detection of shunt stenosis. The reasoning is that after TIPS placement, velocities in the MPV should increase secondary to bypassing the highly resistant intrahepatic portal system. Before TIPS placement, normal MPV velocity is approximately 20 cm/s. After TIPS placement, the velocity measures approximately 40 cm/s.[16,21,22] The Mallinckrodt data used a minimal velocity of 30 cm/s to obtain a sensitivity of 82% and a specificity of 77% in detecting shunt abnormalities. Specifically, in this study, of the 36 patients with MPV velocities less than 30 cm/s, 31 had abnormal venographic results and 5 shunts were normal.[16]

Sonographic Doppler evaluation of the direction of flow within the intrahepatic portal veins is also useful in detecting shunt abnormalities. To reiterate, after placement of a TIPS, the flow in the intrahepatic portal veins should be in the direction of least resistance, which should be toward the functioning stent and away from the liver (hepatofugal). This direction of flow should theoretically reverse (hepatopetal direction) if the stent is stenotic or occluded. This directional change has been studied and shown highly predictive of shunt malfunction but lacks adequate sensitivity.[16,24] The low sensitivity implies that reversal of flow is either difficult to accurately diagnose or is a late manifestation of a stenotic shunt. Moreover, flow within the intrahepatic portal vein branches may fluctuate or differ from day to day and from examination to examination in the normal post-TIPS setting. In the authors' opinion, reversal of flow is a secondary supporting finding and is not the primary indicator of TIPS malfunction. Due to the expected change in direction of portal vein flow (hepatofugal) and the resultant absence of oxygenation via the portal vein branches, the flow in the hepatic arteries should reflexively increase. One study showed that peak systolic arterial velocities increased from 79 cm/s before TIPS placement to 131 cm/s after TIPS placement.[22] This parameter was not statistically significant, however, in the larger study out of Mallinckrodt Institute of Radiology.[16]

Several of the above mentioned Doppler ultrasound parameters, as individual entities, are useful for detecting shunt abnormalities (described previously). As might be predicted, however, when a few of these parameters are combined in interpretation, the sensitivity and specificity both increase. The Mallinckrodt data used 3 criteria to achieve a sensitivity of 92% and a specificity of 72%.[16] The 3 screening criteria they used were abnormal in-stent velocities less than 90 cm/s or greater than 190 cm/s; temporal changes of in-stent velocities, with a decrease of greater than 40 cm/s or an increase greater than 60 cm/s being abnormal; and, finally, portal vein velocity less than 30 cm/s as abnormal.[16] Another large study achieved similar results by combining the velocity measurements, including peak stent velocities, minimum stent velocities, and temporal changes in MPV velocity (sensitivity 94%).[25] Although several of these parameters have proved effective screening criteria, no specific standards exist.

Ultrasound Examination Technique

Considering the technical complexity of the Doppler ultrasound examination itself, radiologists must also have an experienced sonographer who produces accurate results and has a consistent routine. Although technique is often variable from one sonographer to another, consistency and familiarity play an important role in interpretation of Doppler sonography. An agreed-upon sequential imaging protocol may be advisable. Important regions of blood flow that should be evaluated during a Doppler examination include the intrahepatic hepatic veins, the actual stent, the MPV, and intrahepatic portal vein branches. In general, most TIPS are situated deep within the liver and body of the patient and require a low-frequency transducer, such as a 2.5-MHz transducer for adequate visualization. A typical TIPS commonly bridges the right hepatic vein with the right portal vein, which means that the typical hepatic Couinaud segment that is traversed by the TIPS is segment VIII. With any Doppler study, appropriate management of Doppler settings and correct Doppler angle measurements are important. Attention to the phase of respiration is also important for accurate velocity measurements (discussed in detail later).[26]

As with most radiologic modalities, understanding the potential pitfalls and common artifacts is important in accurate interpretation. Simply visualizing the stent under ultrasound can sometimes be difficult, often because of large body habitus and/or a large volume of ascitic fluid. Visualizing the stent and assessing its position should be the first goals of the examination. If blood flow is not detected by conventional color Doppler, power Doppler should be used to assess for any flow in the TIPS. From a technical standpoint, there can be considerable differences in approach and degree of difficulty of a revision of an occluded TIPS compared with a simply narrowed TIPS.

As for assessment of visualized blood flow, attention to gain settings, pulse repetition frequency (PRF), and Doppler angles with the ability to recognize and make adjustments as necessary is important. An inappropriately low or high gain setting can artifactually show absence of flow in a normal stent or presence of flow in an occluded or stenotic stent, respectively.[27] Other potential color Doppler detection errors include an inappropriate adjustment of the PRF. PRF refers to the rate of data sampling and should be adjusted lower to detect slower flow and higher to detect faster flow. In addition, the PRF should be adjusted higher when imaging deeper vessels and vice versa. An image obtained with an inappropriately low PRF may paradoxically show absence of

flow within a normal stent. Conversely if the PRF is set too high, then slower luminal flow may falsely show color aliasing.[27,28] The sonographer must also obtain color ultrasound images with an appropriate Doppler angle. Ideally, the direction of flow within the vessel should form an angle of 45° to 60° with the beam of the transducer for precise velocity measurements. As the Doppler angle approaches 90°, the calculated velocity approaches 0.[27] The difficulty and experience required to obtain velocity measurements with an acceptable Doppler angle on a curved object (TIPS) deep within the abdomen can be imagined.

Velocity measurements can also vary significantly with breathing. One study found velocity measured within the TIPS decreases an average of 22 cm/s during deep inspiration.[26] For this reason, flow velocities should be measured at the end of quiet expiration, if possible. Perhaps more important is simply understanding the differences in flow velocity measurements during the respiratory cycle and making comparisons in similar phases on follow-up examinations. Wachsberg[28] observed a decrease in the MPV velocity at the end of deep inspiration. Furthermore, he describes how it may be easy to obtain an elevated portal vein velocity if the measurement is obtained near the TIPS orifice where there is mixing of the hepatofugal portal vein flow with the splanchnic circulation. To avoid this potential pitfall, the portal vein velocity must be obtained away from the TIPS orifice.[28]

As described previously, the direction of flow within the intrahepatic portal veins and observing directional changes over time can help detect an abnormal stent. Careful analysis of not only the direction but also the spectral tracing is required to accurately identify the intrahepatic portal veins. Unfortunately, intrahepatic portal flow does not follow the expected theoretic direction 100% of the time. One study observed resting hepatopetal flow becoming hepatofugal during deep inspiration.[29] In addition, the same study showed that intrahepatic portal vein flow could change direction when even light pressure was applied to the transducer.[29] The direction of intrahepatic portal vein flow should also be assessed in several regions of the liver because there can be regional changes in flow direction secondary to uneven cirrhotic changes.[24,28] Collateral vessels, specifically, a recanalized paraumbilical vein, can cause the flow within the left portal vein to remain hepatopetal even after TIPS placement whereas the right portal vein should flow in the expected post-TIPS (hepatofugal) direction.[24]

Despite several technical considerations and no widely accepted imaging standardization, hopefully Doppler ultrasound can be seen as a useful tool in screening for TIPS abnormalities in the covered stent era. One study argues, however, that with the superior patency rates of the PTFE-covered stent, long-term screening is not a useful practice.[30] In addition, several other methods for detecting shunt abnormalities have been studied. Studies have shown that CT can be sensitive for detecting significant stenosis, possibly more sensitive and specific than Doppler ultrasound alone.[31,32] Intravenous contrast cannot be given to patients, however, who are significantly allergic to contrast and/or have renal dysfunction. The use of ultrasound contrast agents and even implantable electromechanical pressure sensors has also been studied and had good results but are not widely available.[33,34]

SUMMARY

It should be an interventional radiologist's ultimate responsibility to follow-up, adequately evaluate, and potentially treat a dysfunctional stent. Understanding TIPS anatomy and hemodynamics during and after TIPS placement and reviewing TIPS shunt placement venograms are important to correlate with Doppler ultrasound findings. If a patient with TIPS presents with recurrent symptoms, the patient likely needs an invasive venogram with pressure measurements regardless of the ultrasound results. Ideally, patients do not get to this point, because a recurrence of variceal bleeding may be life threatening. This is why establishing an effective screening test and screening schedule is important. The ideal screening test is Doppler ultrasound. Analyzing abnormal results of the ultrasound parameters (described previously) with subsequent venography and pressure measurements should allow radiologists to gain confidence in interpreting ultrasound TIPS screening examinations.

REFERENCES

1. Ong JP, Sands M, Younossi ZM. Transjugular intrahepatic portosystemic shunts (TIPS): a decade later. J Clin Gastroenterol 2000;30:14–28.
2. Jalan R, Lui HF, Redhead DN, et al. TIPSS 10 years on. Gut 2000;46:578–81.
3. Brown RS Jr, Lake JR. Transjugular intrahepatic portosystemic shunt as a form of treatment for portal hypertension: indications and contraindications. Adv Intern Med 1997;42:485–504.
4. Kerlan RK Jr, LaBerge JM, Gordon RL, et al. Transjugular intrahepatic portosystemic shunts: current status. AJR Am J Roentgenol 1995;164:1059–66.
5. Darcy M. Minimally invasive therapy for portal hypertension. Probl Gen Surg 1999;16:28–43.
6. Coldwell DM, Ring EJ, Rees CR, et al. Multicenter investigation of the role of TIPS shunt in management of portal hypertension. Radiology 1995;196:335–40.
7. Rossle M, Haag K, Ochs A, et al. The transjugular intrahepatic portosystemic stent-shunt for variceal bleeding. N Engl J Med 1994;330:165–71.
8. Laberge JM, Ring EJ, Gordon RL, et al. Creation of TIPS shunts with the Wallstent endoprosthesis: results in 100 patients. Radiology 1993;187:412–20.
9. Nazarian GK, Bjarnason H, Dietz CA Jr, et al. Refractory ascites: midterm results of treatment with a transjugular intrahepatic portosystemic shunt. Radiology 1997;205:173–80.
10. Rossle M, Siegerstetter V, Huber M, et al. The first decade of the transjugular intrahepatic portosystemic shunt (TIPS): state of the art. Liver 1998;18:73–89.
11. Rosado B, Kamath PS. Transjugular intrahepatic portosystemic shunts: an update. Liver Transpl 2003; 9(3):207–17.
12. Haskal ZJ, Pentecost MJ, Soulen MC, et al. Transjugular intrahepatic portosystemic shunt stenosis and revision: early and midterm results. AJR Am J Roentgenol 1994;163:439–44.
13. Haskal ZJ, Carroll JW, Jacobs JE, et al. Sonography of transjugular intrahepatic portosystemic shunts: detection of elevated portosystemic gradients and loss of shunt function. J Vasc Interv Radiol 1997;8: 549–56.
14. Feldstein VA, Patel MD. Doppler ultrasonography of transjugular intrahepatic portosystemic shunts. West J Med 1996;165:56–7.
15. Owens CA, Bartolone C, Warner DL, et al. The inaccuracy of duplex ultrasonography in predicting patency of transjugular intrahepatic portosystemic shunts. Gastroenterology 1998;114:975–80.
16. Kanterman RY, Darcy MD, Middleton WD, et al. Doppler sonography findings associated with transjugular intrahepatic portosystemic shunt malfunction. AJR Am J Roentgenol 1997;168:467–72.
17. Saad WE, Darwish WM, Davies MG, et al. Stent-grafts for transjugular intrahepatic portosystemic shunt creation: Specialized TIPS stent-graft versus generic stent-graft/bare-stent combination. J Vasc Interv Radiol 2010;21:1512–20.
18. Clark TWI, Agaewal R, Haskal ZJ, et al. The effect of initial shunt outflow position on patency of transjugular intrahepatic portosystemic shunt. J Vasc Interv Radiol 2004;15:147–52.
19. Middleton WD, Teefey SA, Darcy MD. Doppler evaluation of transjugular intrahepatic portosystemic shunts. Ultrasound Q 2003;19(2):56–70 [quiz: 108–10].
20. Fung Y, Glajchen N, Shapiro RS, et al. Portal vein velocities measured by ultrasound: usefulness for evaluating shunt function following TIPS placement and TIPS revision. Abdom Imaging 1998;23:511–4.
21. Surratt RS, Middleton WD, Darcy MD, et al. Morphologic and hemodynamic findings at sonography

before and after creation of a transjugular intrahepatic portosystemic shunt. AJR Am J Roentgenol 1993;160:627–30.

22. Foshager MC, Ferral H, Nazarian GK, et al. Duplex sonography after transjugular intrahepatic portosystemic shunts (TIPS): normal hemodynamic findings and efficacy in predicting shunt patency and stenosis. AJR Am J Roentgenol 1995;165:1–7.

23. Dodd GD, Zajko AB, Orons PD, et al. Detection of transjugular intrahepatic portosystemic shunt dysfunction: value of duplex Doppler sonography. AJR Am J Roentgenol 1995;164:1119–24.

24. Lafortune M, Martinet JP, Denys A, et al. Short and long term hemodynamic effects of transjugular intrahepatic portosystemic shunts: a Doppler/manometric correlative study. AJR Am J Roentgenol 1995; 164:997–1002.

25. Zizka J, Elias P, Krajina A, et al. Value of Doppler sonography in revealing transjugular intrahepatic portosystemic shunt malfunction: a 5-year experience in 216 patients. AJR Am J Roentgenol 2000; 175:141–8.

26. Kliewer MA, Hertzberg BS, Henghan JP, et al. Transjugular intrahepatic portosystemic shunts (TIPS): effects of respiratory state and patient position on the measurement of Doppler velocities. AJR Am J Roentgenol 2000;175:149–52.

27. Kruskal J, Newman P, Sammons L, et al. Optimizing doppler and color flow US: application to hepatic sonography. Radiographics 2004;24:657–75.

28. Wachsberg RH. Doppler ultrasound evaluation of transjugular intrahepatic portosystemic shunt function: pitfalls and artifacts. Ultrasound Q 2003;19(3): 139–48.

29. Wachsberg RH, Bahramipour P, Sofocleous CT, et al. Hepatofugal flow in the portal venous system: pathophysiology, imaging findings, and diagnostic pitfalls. Radiographics 2002;22:123–40.

30. Carr C, Tuite C, Soulen MC, et al. Role of ultrasound surveillance of transjugular intrahepatic portosystemic shunts in the covered stent era. J Vasc Interv Radiol 2006;17:1297–305.

31. Chopra S, Dodd G, Chintapalli K, et al. Trans jugular intrahepatic portosystemic shunt: accuracy of helical CT angiography in the detection of shunt abnormalities. Radiology 2000;215:115–22.

32. Fanelli F, Bezzi M, Bruni A, et al. Multidetectorrow computed tomography in the evaluation of transjugular intrahepatic portosystemic shunt performed with expanded-polytetrafluoroethylene-covered stent-graft. Cardiovasc Intervent Radiol 2011;34: 100–5.

33. Uggowitzer MM, Kugler C, Machan L, et al. Value of echo-enhanced Doppler sonography in evaluation of transjugular intrahepatic portosystemic shunts. AJR Am J Roentgenol 1998;170:1041–6.

34. Hirasaki K, Watts J, Suhocki P. Wireless surveillance for transjugular intrahepatic portosystemic shunts (TIPS): a feasibility study. Acad Radiol 2010;17: 418–20.

The Role of Ultrasound in the Preoperative Evaluation, Maturation Process, and Postoperative Evaluation of Hemodialysis Access

Talia Sasson, MD*, Nancy Carson, MBA, RDMS, RVT, Susan Voci, MD

KEYWORDS

• Ultrasound • A-V graft • A-V fistula • Assist maturation • AVF surveillance

KEY POINTS

The goals of this article are as follows:

• Explain why arteriovenous fistulas (AVFs) are the preferred dialysis access method.
• Discuss the challenge of placing fistulas in patient populations that in the past were excluded from this surgery and how ultrasound can help with better patient selection.
• Discuss the maturation process of the AVF and ultrasound's role in early prediction of unsuccessful maturation, which may lead to intervention to salvage the AVF.
• Present the controversies regarding routine surveillance of surgical dialysis access.

 Videos of AVF anastomosis and cephalic vein AVF accompany this article

INTRODUCTION

In 2009, more than 106 000 patients with end-stage renal disease (ESRD) began hemodialysis treatments in the United States, which was an increase of 1.1% from the prior year. The Medicare cost for patients with ESRD in the same year increased 3.1% to a total of $29 billion, which accounted for 5.9% of the Medicare budget.[1] Patients with ESRD may be on hemodialysis for several years while waiting for a renal transplant, and some patients will never receive a transplant.

Therefore, it is imperative that the access for hemodialysis be optimized for each patient.

Hemodialysis is performed either through a central venous dialysis catheter or through permanent surgical access. Surgical access is considered to be superior to dialysis through a central venous dialysis catheter because of reduced complications and costs and increased survival rates of patients. There are 2 types of permanent surgically created hemodialysis access: the native arteriovenous fistula (AVF) and the synthetic arteriovenous graft (AVG). The AVG is a synthetic tube that is surgically

---

Disclosures: There is no financial support provided for this project. The authors have no financial disclosure to report.

Department of Imaging Sciences, University of Rochester Medical Center, 601 Elmwood Avenue, Box 648, Rochester, NY 14642, USA

* Corresponding author.

E-mail address: talia_sasson@urmc.rochester.edu

Ultrasound Clin 8 (2013) 137–146

http://dx.doi.org/10.1016/j.cult.2012.12.003

ultrasound.theclinics.com

anastomosed to an artery and a vein, and the AVF is the direct anastomoses between an artery and a vein. The AVG can be used for dialysis shortly after placement, while the AVF cannot be used for dialysis until it goes through a period of maturation. Despite this delay, once an AVF matures it is associated with a decreased frequency of thrombosis and infection when compared with AVGs. This decrease results in lower hospitalization rates and reduced costs; therefore, the AVF is the preferred method for surgically created hemodialysis.[2] A typical fistula will last 3 years, and an average graft will last less than a year. At some point, most fistulas and grafts will develop a stenosis requiring intervention or revision.[3]

Ultrasound can be used to increase both the success and longevity of surgically created dialysis access. This article reviews the role of ultrasound in each of the following applications: preoperative evaluation (mapping) of the upper extremity veins and arteries, maturation of the AVF, and evaluation of the AVF or AVG for stenosis or thrombosis when dialysis becomes difficult.

ULTRASOUND IN THE PREOPERATIVE EVALUATION OF UPPER EXTREMITY ARTERIES AND VEINS

In an effort to increase the success of AVFs, in 2003 the Centers for Medicaid and Medicare Services and the ESRD networks joined forces to implement the First Breakthrough Initiative, which set an AVF target of 66% of patients undergoing hemodialysis by the year 2009. They have made dramatic progress, effectively promoting the increase in the national AVF prevalence since the program's inception from 32% in May 2003 to nearly 60% in 2011.[4] Although the goal is to increase the percentage of fistulas that reach maturation, without careful planning this aggressive approach to fistula placement may lead to an increase in the number of primary fistula failures caused by thrombosis or inadequate maturation, particularly among patients with marginal vasculature that in the past would have not been considered for AVF placement.[5]

In order for an AVF to reach maturity, it must be created with an artery that can supply enough blood flow to support the access. Blood flow to the limb where the fistula is placed increases considerably, and the artery in that limb must be able to increase in diameter to accommodate the increase in flow. At the same time, the vein that is used for the access should have an adequate size as well as a straight length of at least 10 cm, which allows the placement of 2 needles far enough apart for dialysis. In addition, the vein

should be without areas of stenosis and should be close enough to the skin for needle access.[6,7]

Physical examination is the traditional way for evaluating the suitability of vessels for AVF placement. Evaluation of the upper extremity arteries and veins is performed to assess the arterial and venous diameters, cannulation segment length of the vein, and distance of the vein from the skin surface. Arterial evaluation is also performed to ensure adequate inflow to the fistula.[7] Patients with adequate findings on physical examination seem to achieve similar rates of AVF placement and maturation, although this population makes up only a small percentage of patients undergoing hemodialysis.[6,8]

Preoperative venous and arterial mapping with ultrasound has led to an increase in the number of AVF placements when compared with physical examination evaluation, particularly in patients with inadequate physical examination secondary to obesity, absent pulses, or those with a history of previous access surgeries.[7–9] Another group of patients that can benefit from preoperative ultrasound evaluation are those who are typically considered less suitable for AVF placement, such as older patients or patients with a history of cardiovascular disease or diabetes.[6] Ultrasound is also useful in evaluating suitable veins in the upper arm, such as the basilic vein, which were not routinely used for fistulas in the past.[8–10] Therefore, if physical examination is performed as the initial preoperative evaluation for AVF placement, there needs to be a low threshold for further evaluation with ultrasound before diagnosing patients as unsuitable for AVF placement or not.

The ultrasound performed before AVF creation consists of evaluating both the venous and arterial systems of both arms. A liner transducer with the highest frequency possible should be used to evaluate the lumen of the veins and arteries, usually 9 to 15 MHz. All angle-corrected spectral Doppler tracings are recorded with an angle of insonation of 60° or less to the lumen of the vessel.

The arterial part of the examination is performed first because the venous examination requires the use of a tourniquet, which may affect the arterial flow and arterial spectral waveform characteristics.[2] The examination begins with recording the brachial blood pressures for each arm. Next, the brachial, radial, and ulnar arteries are evaluated with gray scale, color Doppler, and spectral Doppler. The brachial arteries are imaged at the antecubital fossa in the transverse plane to measure the anterior-posterior (AP) diameter and in the sagittal plane to record the angle-corrected peak systolic velocity (Fig. 1). The ulnar and radial arteries are imaged in the transverse and sagittal planes at the levels of

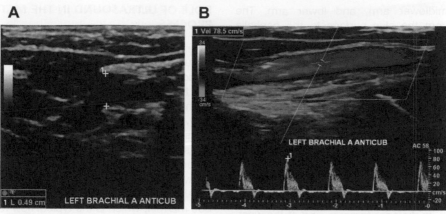

A

B

Fig. 1. Brachial artery evaluation. (*A*) Transverse image of the brachial artery in the antecubital fossa measuring the AP diameter. (*B*) Sagittal color and spectral Doppler image demonstrates the angle-corrected peak systolic velocity equal to 78.5 cm/s.

the midforearm and wrist. The AP diameters and angle-corrected peak velocities are recorded for each site. Calcification of the arteries is documented and classified as mild, moderate, or severe.

For the venous mapping examination, both the superficial and deep veins in each arm are evaluated. Evaluation of the deep system requires documenting patency of the subclavian and axillary veins with gray-scale, color, and spectral Doppler images. The spectral Doppler waveform is an indication of the patency of the central vessels. Diminished pulsatility and respiratory phasicity are considered abnormal and may warrant a closer evaluation of the central vessels before AVF creation.[2] The brachiocephalic vein can be evaluated for patency and waveform characteristics as part of the ultrasound examination by using a small footprint pediatric transducer at the suprasternal notch. Although ultrasound can provide indirect evidence of a central venous lesion, it does not provide direct visualization of the central veins; if there is a history or clinical concern for central

venous stenosis or thrombosis, a venogram should be considered.

Protocols for the evaluation of the superficial veins may vary at each institution. The authors evaluate the cephalic and basilic veins bilaterally in their entirety, thus providing the surgeons with upper extremity mapping. To get maximum venous distention in the superficial veins, it is helpful if patients are sitting or reclining slightly with the arm placed on a bedside table. The room temperature should not be too cool, and patients can be kept warm with blankets, if needed, to ensure maximum venous distention.[2] Starting in the upper arm, a tourniquet is placed as high on the arm as possible. The basilic and cephalic veins of the upper arm are imaged in the transverse plane documenting patency of the vessels with compression and then recording the AP diameter measurement. The measurement is taken by placing the cursors from the anterior wall intima to the posterior wall intima (**Fig. 2**).[2] Images of the cephalic and basilic veins are recorded at the superior arm, superior

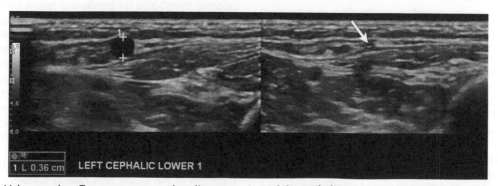

Fig. 2. Vein mapping. Transverse gray-scale split-screen view of the cephalic vein in the upper arm demonstrating a vein diameter of 0.36 cm on the left side of the screen and compressibility of the vein on the right side of the screen (*arrow*).

midarm, midlower arm, and lower arm. The distance from the skin surface to the cephalic vein is also recorded. The cephalic vein may be too deep and difficult to palpate once the AVF has matured if it is greater than 0.5 cm from the skin surface.[11] The tourniquet is removed and the basilic and cephalic veins are followed back to their insertion with the deep system to ensure patency. The tourniquet is then moved to just above the antecubital fossa for evaluation of the lower arm. The cephalic and basilic veins of the forearm are imaged in the transverse plane documenting compression and the AP diameter. Images are recorded in the upper forearm, upper midforearm, midinferior forearm, and at the wrist. It may be necessary to move the tourniquet to the midforearm if veins at the wrist level initially appear too small. The distance of the cephalic vein from the skin surface is also recorded for the forearm. It is not necessary to record the distance of the basilic vein to the skin because if it is used for the fistula, it will be transposed closer to the skin.[2] Minimal transducer pressure should be used when examining the superficial veins because too much pressure will result in vein compression and incorrect AP measurements.

The criteria used to establish vessel size adequacy for fistula placement may vary. According to Silva and colleagues,[12] an arterial diameter greater than 2 mm will increase the rate of AVF maturation. Other investigators have shown that an arterial diameter greater than 1.5 mm should be adequate to support AVF maturation.[13–15] The acceptable venous diameter for AVF placement is considered to be greater than 2.5 mm.[7,12,16]

Some investigators use other criteria, such as the resistive index, to be a good predictor for maturation, especially in women. According to these investigators, the resistive index can assess the ability of the feeding artery to enlarge and adjust to the increased blood flow after fistula placement.[13,17]

As discussed earlier, performing preoperative ultrasound mapping increases the number of AVFs placed, but it is also important to increase the percentage of AVFs that reach adequate maturity. Studies in the literature regarding patients with diabetes and obese patients found that preoperative ultrasound vessel mapping increased the rate of AVF placement and the rate of maturation.[8,18] Women were the only group of patients whereby fistula maturation did not increase when preoperative ultrasound venous mapping was performed.[17]

In summary, preoperative evaluation of the upper extremity with ultrasound mapping increases the rate of AVF placement as well as the rate of maturation in most patients.

ROLE OF ULTRASOUND IN THE MATURATION PROCESS

After an AVF is created, it undergoes a process of maturation. This process involves an increase in blood flow through the artery supplying the fistula and the vein that has been surgically anastomosed to the artery. As a result of the increased blood flow, the diameter of the vein increases and the walls of the vein become thicker, which is referred to as arterialization. At the end of the maturation process, the fistula should be large enough to allow cannulation 3 times a week and to have enough flow to support dialysis at approximately 350 mL/min, which is the typical flow rate used in dialysis centers in the United States.[3,19] Fistulas that do not mature are considered unsuitable for dialysis. Even when preoperative ultrasound mapping is performed, 28% to 53% of fistulas do not mature.[5,20–22] The rate of fistulas that do not mature is higher in the forearm than at the level of the arm.[21]

Assessment for fistula maturity is usually performed clinically by a dialysis nurse or a nephrologist 2 to 3 months after surgery, although some centers will wait up to 6 months for a fistula to mature before declaring it a failure.[5] Clinically, there are certain AVFs that are obviously mature. These AVFs are easily palpable and relatively straight with more than 10-cm length of superficial vein of adequate diameter with a uniform thrill to palpation.[19] It has been shown that an experienced dialysis nurses can predict eventual fistula maturity in 80% of cases.[19] Predicting the outcome of those AVFs that are not clearly mature becomes a problem clinically. This circumstance is when the evaluation with ultrasound becomes important because it can help assess which fistulas will eventually mature and those that may need intervention. Robbin and colleagues,[19] found that a venous diameter of 4 mm or greater and blood flow of 500 mL/min or greater were the optimal thresholds for predicting fistula outcome. In this study, a venous diameter of 4 mm or greater was associated with 89% of fistulas reaching maturation compared with 44% of fistulas that failed to achieve the minimum diameter. Similarly, a blood flow rate of 500 mL or grater was associated with maturation in 84% of fistulas compared with 43% of fistulas with flow rates lower then this threshold. When both size and blood flow rate exceeded the minimum, 94% of the fistulas matured.

Multiple studies suggest that the largest increase in the blood flow rate in fistulas occurs within the first postoperative day and that there is no significant increase in blood flow rate after the first 4 to 6 weeks after surgery. Based on the aforementioned studies, performing an ultrasound examination within the 4- to 6-week postoperative period may be useful in predicting which fistulas are likely to achieve maturation and which fistulas are likely to fail based on vein diameter and flow volume.[15,19,23] This practice would allow early intervention to attempt to salvage an immature fistula that may otherwise go on to fail.

The failure of a fistula to mature may result from one or more anatomic problems, including a stenosis at or near the arteriovenous anastomosis affecting blood flow into the fistula, the presence of one or more large accessory veins directing blood out of the fistula, or a stenosis in the outflow vein. Another potential anatomic problem could result from the vein being too deep for successful cannulation.[24] Ultrasound is an excellent noninvasive means to evaluate anatomic problems that can usually be treated by angioplasty or surgical intervention.

Whether scanning the AVF before maturity or after it has been used for dialysis, the routine is the same. The examination begins with using a high-frequency (9–15 MHz) transducer to perform a transverse gray-scale survey starting with the feeding artery just proximal (cranial) to its anastomosis with the vein. This vein is also referred to as the draining vein, which is actually the AVF. Transverse images are recorded along the feeding artery, anastomotic site, and the draining vein (AVF) to document the presence of any hematomas, fluid collections, intraluminal stenoses, or graft wall pathologic conditions. A hematoma will appear as an area of mixed echogenicity around the lumen or adjacent to the AVF (**Fig. 3**). Often there will be a palpable bump on the extremity.[2] Routine gray-scale measurements of the AVF in the transverse plane consist of the AP diameter of the vein (AVF) and the distance from the anterior vein wall (AVF) to the skin surface at several intervals along the AVF (**Fig. 4**).

Next, interrogation of the artery and AVF in the sagittal plane with gray scale, color, and spectral Doppler is performed. All spectral Doppler tracings are recorded with an angle of 60° or less to the vessel wall. In stenotic areas, the angle correction should be 60° or less to the color jet through the area of stenosis.[11] The imaging sequence should follow the pathway of the actual blood flow beginning with the feeding artery 3 to 4 cm proximal (cranial) to the anastomosis. At this level, gray-scale, color, and angle-corrected spectral Doppler images are recorded. The image sequence of gray scale, color, and angle-corrected spectral Doppler is repeated in the feeding artery 2 cm proximal (cranial) to the anastomosis and at the anastomosis (**Fig. 5**). The peak systolic velocity is recorded for each spectral tracing. The peak systolic velocity (PSV) ratio is then calculated by dividing the PSV at the anastomosis by the PSV obtained in the feeding artery 2 cm cranial to the anastomosis. It has been reported that a PSV ratio of 3.0 or greater indicates a significant stenosis at the anastomosis.[11] Imaging continues through the draining vein (AVF) in the sagittal plane with gray scale, color, and spectral Doppler. The typical flow pattern of the AVF is generally high velocity, with low-resistance characteristics (high diastolic flow and pulsatile) (**Fig. 6**). An angle-corrected velocity is recorded from within the AVF just distal to the anastomosis, which is the inferior or caudal part of the AVF. Sagittal imaging of the AVF and venous runoff continues all the way back to the subclavian vein. If the AVF appears narrowed at any point, an angle-corrected PSV is recorded at the narrowing and 2 cm distal to the narrowing. A PSV ratio can be calculated by dividing the PSV at the stenotic area by the PSV 2 cm distal to the stenotic area. If the ratio is 2.0 or greater, the stenotic area is classified as a 50% or greater diameter narrowing.[11]

At some institutions, actual blood flow is record in the AVF. This measurement is obtained in an

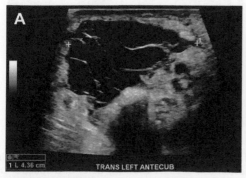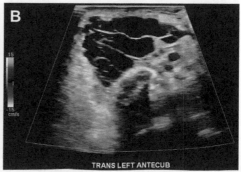

Fig. 3. Hematoma. Gray-scale (*A*) and color Doppler (*B*) images demonstrating a hematoma in the antecubital fossa measuring 4.36 cm.

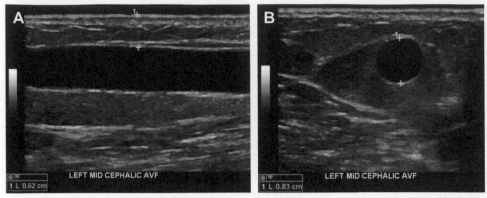

Fig. 4. AVF. (*A*) Sagittal gray-scale image at mid AVF demonstrating the distance from the skin surface to the AVF equal to 0.62 cm. (*B*) Transverse gray-scale image at mid AVF measuring the diameter of the fistula equal to 0.83 cm.

area of the AVF that is fairly straight where the walls can be imaged in parallel, at least 10 cm from the anastomosis.[14] Using the highest frequency possible and the heel-toe method, a Doppler angle of 60° or less to the vessel wall must first be achieved. The Doppler sample gate is opened to include the entire vessel but not overextending the vessel wall. At least 3 cardiac waveforms are captured to estimate the time-averaged mean velocity. The internal diameter of the vessel is then measured and the calculation package on the machine calculates the volume of blood flow: time average mean velocity multiplied by the vessel cross-sectional area.[11] It is recommended that 3 flow measurements be obtained as described.[2]

The AVF is also evaluated for large branches, which are most important when found in the first 10 cm from the anastomosis. These veins can actually divert from the AVF, which may prolong or prevent the maturing process or decrease the AVF flow below the desired level for successful dialysis.[11]

The examination is concluded by imaging the feeding artery just distal (caudal) to the anastomosis. Here an angel-corrected spectral Doppler tracing is recorded to document the direction of flow. The radial and ulnar arteries are also evaluated at the level of the wrist documenting direction of flow with color Doppler and angle-corrected spectral Doppler. It is common for the direction of the radial artery to be reversed (radial steal), but patients will not be symptomatic (**Fig. 7**). Steal syndrome is a situation when after the placement of dialysis access, patients actually develop symptoms of distal limb ischemia secondary to the inability of the artery to supply enough blood flow to both the AFV (or AVG) and the distal limb. In this situation, enough blood is being diverted from the hand back to the AVF or AVG causing ischemic symptoms, which can be treated if severe enough.[2]

In summary, ultrasound surveillance of the maturing fistula, when done 4 to 6 weeks after

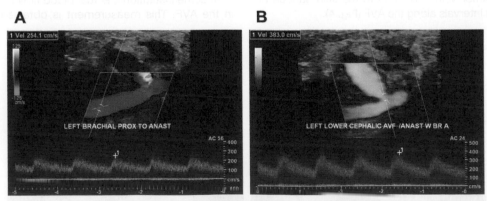

Fig. 5. Brachial artery to AVF anastomosis. (*A*) Sagittal color and spectral Doppler image demonstrating the velocity of the brachial artery 2 cm proximal to the anastomosis is 254.1 cm/s. (*B*) Color and spectral Doppler image of the anastomosis, the angle-corrected velocity is 383.0 cm/s. The PSV ratio of the anastomosis to the brachial artery 2 cm proximal to the anastomosis is equal to 1.5, which is normal.

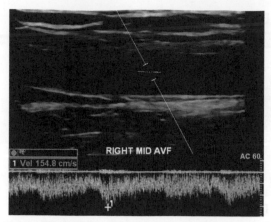

Fig. 6. AVF flow. Sagittal spectral Doppler image of the midportion of an AVF demonstrating the normal AVF flow pattern, high velocity, pulsatile, and high diastolic flow.

surgery, can successfully predict maturation and, in most cases, diagnose the anatomic problems, which may prevent maturation of the fistula. In many cases, the correction of these problems by endovascular or surgical means can salvage the immature fistula (**Fig. 8**). Singh and colleagues[25] showed that 78% of sonographically immature fistulas that underwent a procedure or surgery to correct the anatomic problem diagnosed by ultrasound went on to mature and were used successfully for dialysis. By comparison, only 31% of fistulas in which ultrasound diagnosed a problem and no salvage procedure was performed could eventually be used for dialysis.

ROLE OF ULTRASOUND IN MONITORING AVFS AND GRAFTS

As discussed in the introduction, AVFs are considered to be superior to grafts because of a decreased

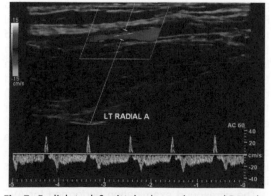

Fig. 7. Radial steal. Sagittal color and spectral Doppler image of the radial artery at the level of the wrist. Both color and spectral demonstrate flow direction away from the hand.

frequency of thrombosis, infection, and pseudoaneurysm formation, as well as increased longevity. Despite this, most fistulas and grafts will develop a stenosis at some point, requiring intervention or revision. Once an access is thrombosed, its longevity will be shorter than if the underlying lesion had been treated before the development of a thrombus. Therefore, detecting the underlying lesion (stenosis) before thrombus formation is essential.

Monitoring and surveillance of fistulas and grafts can be performed by physical examination, measurement of static venous pressures and flow during dialysis access, and by a formal ultrasound examination. Clinical evaluation of the fistula or graft can be performed at the time of dialysis looking for signs of malfunction, such as a reduced thrill, difficulty with cannulation, palpation of a mass, or prolonged bleeding after needles are removed. The kidney disease outcomes quality initiative guidelines currently endorse the measurement of static venous pressures once monthly. If elevated, this would indicate an outflow stenosis. Another recommendation is to measure the flow in the dialysis access as an indirect sign of a problem.[26] Both measurements have been reported as inaccurate.[27]

In an effort to prevent thrombosis and increase the longevity of AVFs and AVGs, several prospective studies were performed to assess the role of ultrasound surveillance in addition to clinical monitoring. The studies that evaluated AVGs found that ultrasound surveillance did find more significant (greater than 50%) stenoses compared with clinical assessment alone, which also resulted in more angioplasties. The studies did not, however, find a decrease in the rate of thrombosis; there was no increase in the long-term patency of the grafts.[28,29] When considering ultrasound surveillance and early treatment of AVFs, most studies performed found that ultrasound surveillance may decrease thrombosis in AVFs but it does not increase longevity of the fistula.[30] Although ultrasound surveillance of AVFs may not improve longevity, it has been reported that it does contribute to the reduction in use of central venous dialysis catheters and their associated complications, which ultimately reduces hospitalization costs.[31]

The ultrasound examination performed for graft surveillance is very similar to the examination performed for the AVF. The synthetic graft is easily imaged because of the echogenic appearance of the graft walls on ultrasound (**Fig. 9**). This examination also begins with a transverse gray-scale survey starting with the feeding artery just proximal (cranial) to its anastomosis with graft. Transverse images are recorded along the feeding artery, at the arterial anastomosis, within the graft, at the venous anastomosis, and within the draining vein

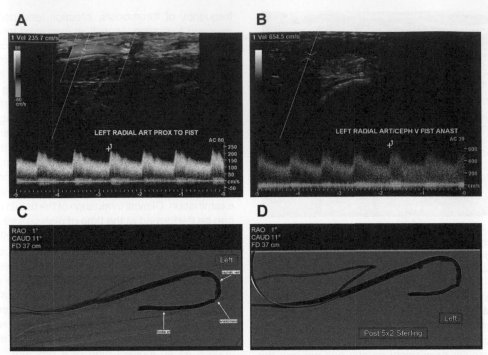

Fig. 8. Confirmed Cimino AVF stenosis with intervention. (*A*) Four weeks after surgery, spectral Doppler demonstrates the radial artery 2 cm cephalic to the anastomosis measures 235.7 cm/s. (*B*) Angle-corrected spectral Doppler demonstrating the velocity at the anastomosis is greater than 654.5 cm/s. The ratio is at least 2.8, which was reported as stenotic. (*C*) Fistulogram showing a stenosis in the arteriovenous anastomosis and a small cephalic vein. (*D*) Follow-up examination showing normal anastomosis and considerable increase in diameter of the cephalic vein.

documenting the presence of any hematomas, fluid collections, intraluminal stenosis, or graft wall pathologic condition. The only additional complication to be aware of is the potential pseudoaneurysm, which may result from the actual needle punctures during dialysis. A pseudoaneurysm will look like a mass outside of the lumen of the AVF; but color Doppler inside of the pseudoaneurysm will show an aliasing pattern, and spectral Doppler will be characteristic of a yin/yang flow pattern (**Fig. 10**). Every effort should be made to find the neck of the pseudoaneurysm, which is where it comes off of the graft.

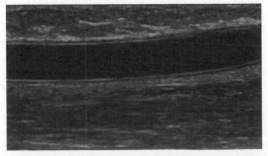

Fig. 9. AVG. Sagittal gray-scale image of an AVG demonstrating the echogenic parallel lines, which represent the walls of the graft.

Sagittal gray-scale, color, and spectral Doppler images are recorded at the same locations. Peak systolic velocities are recorded 2 cm proximal (cranial) to the arterial anastomosis, at the arterial anastomosis, within the graft 2 cm distal to the arterial anastomosis, midgraft, 2 cm proximal to the venous anastomosis, and at the venous anastomosis. The typical flow pattern of the graft is also high velocity, with low-resistance characteristics (high diastolic flow and pulsatile). If the graft appears narrowed at any point, an angle-corrected PSV is recorded at the narrowing and 2 cm distal to the narrowing. The PSV ratios are calculated the same way as for the fistula. The draining vein is then followed all the way to the subclavian vein to ensure patency. The examination is concluded by imaging the feeding artery just distal (caudal) to the anastomosis and the radial and ulnar arteries.

The most common site of graft stenosis is at the anastomosis of the graft with the draining vein, followed by within the graft; the arterial anastomosis is the least likely area for stenosis.[2]

The ultrasound examination performed for AVF surveillance is essentially the same as that performed when evaluating for AVF maturity. The only additional finding to be aware of is the potential

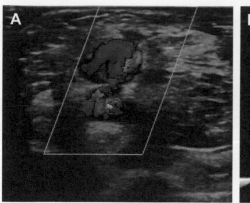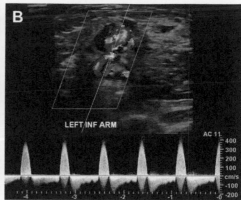

Fig. 10. Pseudoaneurysm. (*A*) Transverse color Doppler image of a pseudoaneurysm in the arm demonstrating color Doppler aliasing. (*B*) Spectral Doppler indicating the yin/yang flow pattern of the pseudoaneurysm.

pseudoaneurysm, as was described with graft surveillance.

In summary, the role of routine ultrasound surveillance of fistulas and grafts is at best controversial; however, as discussed, ultrasound does have an important role in the further evaluation of potential problems found clinically. When ultrasound was compared with a fistulogram in diagnosing stenoses in both fistulas (AVFs) and grafts (AVGs), it was found to be both accurate and sensitive.[32,33] Surveillance ultrasounds are also very helpful when an AVG or AVF requires intervention, specifically in planning for the cannulation site and reducing the number of cannulations required per procedure, reducing the actual procedure time, thus, reducing the radiation dose.[32,33]

SUMMARY

Ultrasound is a relatively inexpensive and readily available tool that contributes to the successful placement and maintenance of dialysis access. In the preoperative stage, ultrasound mapping helps by increasing the number of AVFs placed by finding suitable veins that are not easily assessed by physical examination. Once the AVF is placed, ultrasound surveillance of the fistula 4 to 6 weeks after surgery detects which fistulas are not likely to mature; these patients can be referred for early intervention to salvage the fistula. The role of ultrasound in routine surveillance of fistulas and graft is controversial, but using ultrasound to diagnose a stenosis once a clinical problem accrues does enable the interventionist to better choose his or her approach to the procedure.

VIDEOS

Videos related to this article can be found online at http://dx.doi.org/10.1016/j.cult.2012.12.003.

REFERENCES

1. U.S. Renal Data System. USRDS 2011 annual data report: atlas of chronic kidney disease and end-stage renal disease in the United States. Bethesda (MD): National Institutes of Health, National Institute of Diabetes and Digestive and Kidney Diseases; 2011.
2. Umphrey HR, Lockhart ME, Abts CA, et al. Dialysis grafts and fistulae: planning and assessment. Ultrasound Clin 2011;6:477–89.
3. Wilson SE. Vascular access: principles and practice. Philadelphia: Lippincott Williams & Wilkins; 2010. 5th edition, Chapter 12.
4. Vassalotti JA, Jennings WC, Beathard GA, et al, Fistula First Breakthrough Initiative Community Education Committee. Fistula first breakthrough initiative: targeting catheter last in fistula first. Semin Dial 2012;25(3):303–10.
5. Allon M, Lockhart ME, Lilly RZ, et al. Effect of preoperative sonographic mapping on vascular access outcomes in hemodialysis patients. Kidney Int 2001; 60:2013–20.
6. Ferring M, Henderson J, Wilmink A, et al. Vascular ultrasound for the preoperative evaluation prior to arteriovenous fistula formation for hemodialysis: review of the evidence. Nephrol Dial Transplant 2008;23(6): 1809–15.
7. Asif A, Ravani P, Roy-Chaudhury P, et al. Vascular mapping techniques: advantages and disadvantages. J Nephrol 2007;20:299–303.
8. Patel ST, Hughes J, Mills JL. Failure of arteriovenous fistula maturation: an unintended consequence of exceeding dialysis outcome quality initiative guidelines for hemodialysis access. J Vasc Surg 2003; 38(3):439–49.
9. Kakkos SK, Haddad GK, Stephanou A, et al. Routine preoperative venous and arterial mapping increases both construction and maturation rate of upper arm autogenous arteriovenous fistulae. Vasc Endovascular Surg 2011;45(2):135–41.

10. Karakayali F, Ekici Y, Gorur SK, et al. The value of preoperative vascular imaging in the selection and success of hemodialysis access. Ann Vasc Surg 2007;21(4):481–9.

11. Robbin ML, Lockhart ME. Ultrasound evaluation before and after hemodialysis access. In: Pellerito J, Polak JF, editors. Introduction to vascular ultrasonography. 6th edition. Philadelphia: Elsevier; 2012. p. 281–93.

12. Silva MB Jr, Hobson RW, Pappas PJ, et al. A strategy for increasing use of autogenous hemodialysis access procedures: impact of preoperative noninvasive evaluation. J Vasc Surg 1998;27:302–7.

13. Malovrh M. Non-invasive evaluation of vessels by duplex sonography prior to construction of arteriovenous fistulas for hemodialysis. Nephrol Dial Transplant 1998;13:125–9.

14. Parmar J, Aslam M, Standfield N. Pre-operative radial arterial diameter predicts early failure of arteriovenous fistula (AVF) for hemodialysis. Eur J Vasc Endovasc Surg 2007;33:113–5.

15. Wong V, Ward R, Taylor J, et al. Factors associated with early failure of arteriovenous fistulae for hemodialysis access. Eur J Vasc Endovasc Surg 1996;12:207–13.

16. Lauvao LS, Ihnat DM, Goshima KR, et al. Vein diameter is the major predictor of fistula maturation. J Vasc Surg 2009;49(6):1499–504.

17. Lockhart ME, Robbin ML, Allon M. Preoperative sonographic radial artery evaluation and correlation with subsequent radiocephalic fistula outcome. J Ultrasound Med 2004;23:161–8.

18. Sedlacek M, Teodorescu V, Falk A, et al. Hemodialysis access placement with preoperative noninvasive vascular mapping: comparison between patients with and without diabetes. Am J Kidney Dis 2001;38(3):560–4.

19. Robbin ML, Chamberlain NE, Lockhart ME, et al. Hemodialysis arteriovenous fistula maturity: US evaluation. Radiology 2002;225(1):59–64.

20. Palder SB, Kirkman RL, Whittemore AD, et al. Vascular access for hemodialysis: patency rates and results of revision. Ann Surg 1985;202:235–9.

21. Miller PE, Tolwani A, Luscy CP, et al. Predictors of adequacy of arteriovenous fistulas in hemodialysis patients. Kidney Int 1999;56:275–80.

22. Won T, Jang JW, Lee S, et al. Effects of intraoperative blood flow on the early patency of radiocephalic fistulas. Ann Vasc Surg 2000;14:468–72.

23. Lomonte C, Casucci F, Antonelli M, et al. Is there a place for duplex screening of the brachial artery in the maturation of arteriovenous fistulas? Semin Dial 2005;18(3):243–6.

24. Allon M, Robbin ML. Increasing arteriovenous fistulas in hemodialysis patients: problems and solutions. Kidney Int 2002;62(4):1109–24.

25. Singh P, Robbin ML, Lockhart ME, et al. Clinically immature arteriovenous hemodialysis fistulas: effect of US on salvage. Radiology 2008;246:299–305.

26. National Kidney Foundation: KDOQI clinical practice guidelines for vascular access, update 2000. Am J Kidney Dis 2001;37(Suppl 1):S137–81.

27. Paulson WD, Moist L, Lok CE. Vascular access surveillance: an ongoing controversy. Kidney Int 2012;81:132–42. Kidney Dis 1999;34:478–85.

28. Ram SJ, Work J, Caldito GC, et al. A randomized controlled trial of blood flow and stenosis surveillance of hemodialysis grafts. Kidney Int 2003;64: 272–80.

29. Robbin ML, Oser RF, Lee JY, et al. Randomized comparison of ultrasound surveillance and clinical monitoring on arteriovenous graft outcomes. Kidney Int 2006;69:730–5.

30. Tonelli M, James M, Wiebe N, et al. Ultrasound monitoring to detect access stenosis in hemodialysis patients: a systematic review. Am J Kidney Dis 2008;51:630–40.

31. Work J. Role of access surveillance and preemptive intervention. Semin Vasc Surg 2011;24(2):137–42.

32. Doelman C, Duijm LE, Liem YS, et al. Stenosis detection in failing hemodialysis access fistulas and grafts: comparison of color Doppler ultrasonography, contrast-enhanced magnetic resonance angiography, and digital subtraction angiography. J Vasc Surg 2005;42(4):739–46.

33. Dumars MC, Thompson WE, Bluth EI, et al. Management of suspected hemodialysis graft dysfunction: usefulness of diagnostic US. Radiology 2002;222: 103–7.

Ultrasound-Guided Solid-Organ Biopsy

Thomas LoStracco, MD, Refky Nicola, MS, DO*,
Labib Syed, MD, MPH

KEYWORDS

- Percutaneous biopsy • Ultrasound • Kidney • Liver • Spleen • Bleeding

KEY POINTS

- Appropriate indications for ultrasound-guided solid-organ biopsy are discussed.
- Preprocedural and postprocedural patient care is outlined.
- An ultrasound-guided technique to obtain an adequate core specimen from the liver, kidney, and spleen is described.
- New techniques and technology to facilitate ultrasound-guided solid-organ biopsy are introduced.

INTRODUCTION

As sophisticated as medical imaging has become, the technology has not yet reached the point at which a diagnosis can be established based on imaging alone. Samples of tissue or cells are still relied on to establish a definitive diagnosis. To obtain a sample, ultrasound, computed tomography (CT), and magnetic resonance (MR) imaging are used as safe and effective means of image guidance when performing a biopsy.[1] This article focuses on ultrasound-guided biopsy of solid abdominal organs, with emphasis on preprocedural preparation and technique. Examples are provided to show the technique using the appropriate ultrasound settings, transducers, and needles safely to obtain an adequate specimen from the liver, kidney, and spleen.

CT provides better spatial resolution for biopsying lesions within smaller organs, as well as in organs without the appropriate acoustic medium, such as bone, bowel, and lung. Recent advances in MR imaging guidance also provide excellent spatial resolution without ionizing radiation, although the length of the procedure and associated cost may be prohibitive. However, ultrasonography has the benefit of providing real-time images

for immediate feedback, which is especially advantageous when advancing the needle. It also has the benefit of avoiding ionizing radiation and lowering the cost and expenditure of a department's resources, compared with CT or MR imaging.[2] Therefore, in larger abdominal organs, such as the liver, kidneys, and spleen, ultrasonography can be the modality of choice for image-guided solid-organ biopsy. However, the use of ultrasonography requires skill and is operator dependent. In this article, technique is discussed, as well as preprocedural and postprocedural care for patients undergoing ultrasound-guided biopsy of the solid organs.

HISTORY

The term biopsy originates from Greek and means "to see life." It was coined by the French dermatologist, Ernest Besnier, in 1879,[3] who used the term to describe skin samples from his patients. In 1883, Erlich[4] performed the first liver aspiration. Then, in 1923, he performed the first percutaneous liver biopsy for diagnostic purposes.

The first open renal biopsy was performed in 1901. The first radiography-guided percutaneous biopsy was performed in 1944 by Nils Alwall[5]

The authors have no financial disclosures.
Division of Interventional Radiology, Department of Imaging Sciences, University of Rochester Medical Center, PO Box 648, Rochester, NY 14642, USA
* Corresponding author.
E-mail address: refky_nicola@urmc.rochester.edu

Ultrasound Clin 8 (2013) 147–154
http://dx.doi.org/10.1016/j.cult.2012.12.010
1556-858X/13/$ – see front matter Published by Elsevier Inc.

and described in the literature by Iversen and Braun in 1951.[6] These biopsies were performed using intravenous (IV) pyelography. In 1954, Kark and Meuhrcke[7] described the use of a cutting Vim-Silverman needle with patients in the prone position. Goldberg and colleagues[8] described ultrasound-guided renal biopsy in 1975. However, the technique used for solid-organ biopsy[8] has gradually evolved, as medical imaging has become more advanced.

INDICATIONS

Biopsy may be performed to randomly obtain tissue from an organ, such as in a patient with diffuse parenchymal disease, or to analyze a specific lesion within the organ that was discovered on a previous imaging study. This situation depends on the patient's history and previous studies. Because biopsy collects tissue, this yields crucial information not only about the diagnosis but also about the stage of the disease process. Biopsy may be the only means of obtaining a diagnosis. The common indications for liver biopsy are listed in **Box 1**.[4] In addition, the indications for kidney biopsy are listed in **Box 2**.[9–11]

PREPROCEDURAL CARE

Although there are numerous indications for a solid-organ biopsy, more often it is requested to evaluate for mass. The biopsy can be distressing and a source of anxiety for a patient. It is the responsibility of the interventional radiologist to explain the indication completely, as well as the risks, benefits, and alternatives of the procedure in terms that the patient understands so that they can make an informed decision before the procedure.

Box 1
Indications for liver biopsy
Acute and chronic hepatitis
After liver transplant
Iron and copper metabolism abnormalities
Glycogen storage disorders
Tuberculosis
Primary biliary cirrhosis
Hepatocellular carcinoma
Focal nodular hyperplasia
Metastases
Hemangioma

Box 2
Indications for renal biopsy
Solid masses
Confirmation of suspected renal cell carcinoma (RCC) when surgical risk is high
Confirmation of suspected RCC when disease is locally advanced or metastatic
Diagnosis of a renal mass with equivocal imaging features
Diagnosis of a renal mass in a solitary or transplant kidney
Diagnosis of a renal mass in a patient with extrarenal malignancy
Complex cystic masses
After renal transplant
Acute kidney injury (not explained by hypoperfusion or outlet obstruction)
Nephrotic syndrome
Proteinuria of unknown cause
Systemic disease affecting the kidneys
Systemic lupus erythematosus
Wegener granulomatosis
Goodpasture syndrome
Human immunodeficiency virus

The process begins with contacting the patient at least 1 week before the procedure, if the biopsy is being performed on an outpatient basis. They should be informed about which medication they need to discontinue and for how long; this information is listed in **Table 1**.[12] Patients need to be informed that they are to remain nil-by-mouth after midnight on the day of the procedure, or at least 8 hours before, if they are to receive conscious (moderate) sedation. When the patient comes to the hospital, a complete clinical history-taking and focused physical examination should be

Table 1		
Medication discontinuance in preparation for biopsy		
Medication		**Discontinue (Before Procedure)**
Antiplatelets		5–7 d
Warfarin		5 d
Unfractionated heparin		1 6 h
Low-molecular-weight heparin		24 h

performed. All medications and allergies should be recorded in the medical record and reviewed to ensure that there are no drug interactions, adverse reactions, or allergic reactions once the patient receives sedation.

Laboratory workup is necessary to determine the patient's risk for bleeding or other complications. This workup includes platelet count, prothrombin time/international normalized ratio (INR), and partial thromboplastin time. At our institution, a platelet count of less than 50,000 or an INR of greater than 1.5 is a contraindication for proceeding with the biopsy. In these cases, administration of platelets and fresh frozen plasma, respectively, can be considered depending on the clinical situation. In addition to fresh frozen plasma, vitamin K can be also be administered for an increased INR. Values should be rechecked before the procedure to ensure that they are within the appropriate range. Normal values do not necessarily preclude postprocedural bleeding. In addition, at our institution, we also obtain a glomerular filtration rate on patients who are undergoing renal biopsy to determine the underlying kidney function.

Because solid-organ biopsy is an invasive procedure, moderate sedation is used to provide adequate patient comfort for the procedure. If there are no contraindications, we use fentanyl (Sublimaze) and midazolam (Versed), 200 μg and 1 mg, respectively. The doses must be adjusted accordingly for age, weight, tolerance to anxiolytics or opiates, as well as vital signs. If the patient has not remained nil-by-mouth for the allotted time, only 1 of the moderate sedation agents, either fentanyl can be used to safely keep the patient comfortable through the procedure.[13] Once the patient is in the suite, a time out or a dedicated pause should be observed by the interventional radiologist, technologist, nurse, and any other individual involved in the case, to recheck patient identification and the procedure to be performed, before proceeding.

Besides coagulopathy, contraindications to liver biopsy include an uncooperative patient, encephalopathy, hepatic failure with severe jaundice, and serious systemic disease. Extrahepatic obstruction and bacterial cholangitis are also contraindications, which may both lead to peritonitis and septicemia. A large ascites may complicate access to the liver for biopsy, but are not considered a contraindication. A paracentesis can be performed before biopsy.[4] Contraindications to renal biopsy include an uncooperative patient, uncontrolled hypertension (systolic blood pressure >180 mm Hg), renal or perirenal infection, solitary kidney, small (<9 cm in longitudinal axis) and echogenic native kidneys.[14]

POSTPROCEDURAL CARE
Patient Monitoring

After the procedure, patients are escorted to the recovery area for continuous monitoring of vital signs, oxygen saturation, and pain scale. At our institution, patients are monitored intensely for the first 3 hours after the procedure and are instructed to remain in bed until the 3 hours have elapsed. Also, the site of access is assessed periodically for signs of bleeding or evolving hematoma. As a precaution, patients are instructed to lie in a right lateral decubitus position, left lateral decubitus position, or supine depending on the site of entry to apply pressure to the entry site.[15]

During the first hour, patients are restricted from eating and drinking and IV access is maintained. However, IV fluids are administered until oral intake is initiated. Afterward, their diet is advanced as tolerated. This strategy is particularly important in patients who have been given conscious sedation.

Discharge and Follow-Up Instructions

Before the patient is discharged, a complete assessment of their vital signs, mental status, ability to eat, drink, void, and walk, pain scale, and bleeding at the puncture site is made by the nursing staff. If the patient is deemed stable, then they are permitted to leave in the company of an adult. Specific discharge instructions are given to patients to return to the hospital if their condition worsens or they are experiencing increasing pain or weakness in the area. Patients who have received conscious sedation are instructed to avoid operating any heavy machinery or driving a car for 24 hours. Within a few days after the procedure, patients are informed to follow up with their referring physicians, who will discuss the results of the procedure and the next appropriate steps.

For any type of ultrasound-guided biopsy, a wide variety of needles are available to the operator. These needles are divided into groups based on gauge (size), tip configuration, and mechanism of sample acquisition. In most cases, size is the most important determinant in choosing a needle. Broadly, needle size can be placed in 2 categories: smaller size encompasses 20 to 25 gauge, whereas the larger size encompasses 14 to 19 gauge. In general, the smaller sizes are used for superficial parts, such as thyroid, or when the risk of bleeding is accentuated, such as splenic biopsy. The larger sizes are preferred when core samples are required. Smaller-gauge needles can provide adequate cytologic material and some histologic material. They can minimize bleeding, especially if multiple passes are required. The major downside to these needles is the difficulty in directing them because of their thinness. Conversely, larger needles are easier to direct and provide better samples for cytology and histology, with fewer needle passes. The drawback with these needles is the increased risk of bleeding.

Needles may also be classified by tip configuration. The most common breakdown is between noncutting and cutting types. The noncutting needles such as Chiba and spinal are known as aspiration needles, whereas cutting needles such as Westcott and Greene can be further subdivided into end-cut and side-cut types. Each of these needles can also vary in the angle and bevel of the tip. The Chiba and spinal needles have bevel angles of 25° and 30°, respectively, whereas the Westcott and Greene have 90° tips. Needle manufacturers are offering both needles and needle tips with an echogenic coating to increase visibility with ultrasonography. This coating has proved to be significantly better in needle visualization in phantoms with ultrasonography.

When a specific lesion is targeted, particularly a smaller lesion, precise measurement is imperative in choosing a needle size. The throw of the biopsy needle should reflect the size of the lesion. Most of the cutting-type needles used for visceral core biopsies are spring loaded and make a clicking noise when deployed. We routinely fire the biopsy needle before usage so the patient is accustomed to the click sound.

Liver Biopsy

Using an ultrasound machine with Doppler capability and a 4-MHz to 5-MHz transducer, the liver is assessed for the best possible approach, whether it is for a focal mass or to obtain a random sample. At our institution, we use the transducer guide bracket with the ultrasound probe to facilitate needle entry. A sterile tray is prepared. The contents of the tray usually contain 10 to 20 mL of 1% lidocaine, 4 × 4 sterile gauges, sterile saline, sterile Q-tips, 21-gauge infiltration needle, spinal needle, and 11-blade incision scalpel. The area is prepared and draped in sterile fashion.[16]

For a random liver biopsy, our ideal approach is the subcostal because of the elevated positioning of the diaphragm and pleura. However, in most cases, an intercostal approach is taken to target the posterior right lobe of the liver and thus avoid surrounding structures such as lung, pleura, colon, stomach, gallbladder, and vascular structures. The intercostal approach between the 10th and 11th rib is the preferred method of entry.[17] The transducer is placed at the interspace such that the acoustic shadowing of the lung can be visualized superiorly and the needle placed inferiorly (**Fig. 1**). When using the intercostal approach, great care must be taken to avoid the neurovascular bundle coursing along the inferior margin of the rib. One technique is to inject 1% lidocaine generously at the inferior costal margin, which pushes the neurovascular bundle superiorly and out of the anticipated tract of the needle. If the right lobe is not an option or there is a mass in the left lobe, the most lateral segment of the left lobe is recommended. Ultrasound with color Doppler is used to assess the surrounding vascular structures (**Fig. 2**).

The biopsy of a transplanted liver is performed to assess for signs of rejection, both early and late stage, preservation-perfusion injury, recurrent disease, or cytomegalovirus. Biopsy can be performed in the early stage (eg, within 7 days) or in the late stages (within 6 months).[18]

The skin is anesthetized with 1% lidocaine. Afterward, a 22-gauge needle is used to inject lidocaine deeper into the liver capsule before insertion of the biopsy needle. With an 11-blade incision scalpel, a small incision in the skin is made. At our institution, we prefer to use a coaxial 19-gauge needle or 18-gauge biopsy needle through the transducer guide bracket.[19] The benefits of the coaxial system are that multiple passes are allowed without losing

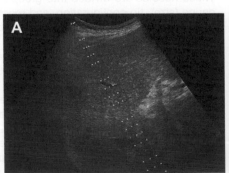
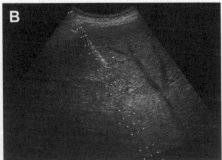

Fig. 1. (*A, B*) Two transverse grayscale images of the liver, showing image guidance of a random liver biopsy.

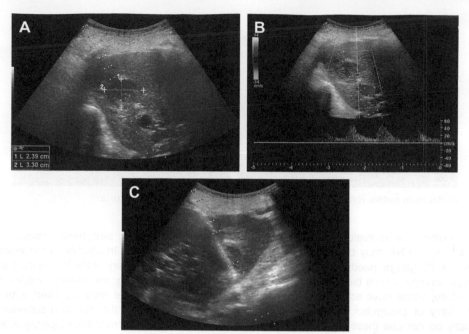

Fig. 2. (*A*) Grayscale image showing a hypoechoic mass at the dome of the liver. (*B*) Color and spectral Doppler ultrasonography of an arterial vessel at the outer margin of the mass. (*C*) Needle passing through the center of the lesion to avoid the vessel.

position and only a single puncture is made into the hepatic capsule. This procedure reduces the risk of bleeding and seeding from the needle.[20] About 2 or 3 passes are performed. After the procedure is complete, 3 or 4 Gelfoam (Ethicon, Sommerville, NJ, USA) pledgets or Gelfoam mixture are injected into the track through the coaxial needle.[21] This technique has been shown to reduce the incidents of bleeding or progression of bleeding. When targeting a focal lesion, a needle trajectory is chosen to include a portion of normal liver tissue. This approach aids with the tamponade effect if there is bleeding from the target lesion and may also prevent seeding.[19]

Kidney Biopsy

Essentially, the same medications, materials, and equipment are used when performing an ultrasound-guided renal biopsy. However, the patient's positioning and approach are modified according to the position of the mass. The shortest and most accessible trajectory is performed, avoiding injury to surrounding organs. If the indication is for a nonfocal lesion, at our institution, patients are typically placed in the left lateral decubitus position to splint the normal motion of the left kidney with respiration. The lower pole is the preferred location because it is a less vascular location.[22] The needle is positioned from a posterior approach along the posterior axillary line to

avoid surrounding organs.[4] For nonfocal renal cortical biopsies, the lower pole is once again selected. Usually, the left kidney is targeted because it is lower than the right. The needle is placed tangentially to capture the cortex and avoid the medullary and collecting systems (**Fig. 3**).[23]

Certain modifications with position and approach are necessary in patients with a focal lesion or a renal transplant. If the indication is for a focal mass, having the patient in the prone lateral decubitus position may facilitate access. Typically, the transplanted kidney is placed in the right or left lower pelvis, thus the supine position is the best means of access, with an anterior approach as the shortest distance (**Fig. 4**). It is recommended that Doppler ultrasound be used to avoid adjacent vascular structures. The most common indication similar to biopsy of kidney transplant is to assess for allograft rejection.[24] When performing the biopsy, it is recommended to avoid any peritransplant fluid collections, to reduce the risk of bleeding and infection. If there is a mass within the allograft, it may represent posttransplant lymphoproliferative disorder, which also requires a core biopsy and flow cytometry for further analysis.[2]

Either fine-needle aspiration (FNA) or core biopsy can be performed. At our institution, we prefer a core biopsy using a 17-gauge coaxial needle within an ultrasound transducer guide bracket with an 18-gauge core biopsy needle with 2 or 3 passes.[20] The specimen is then analyzed by an

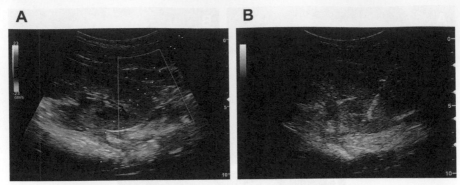

Fig. 3. (A, B) Random native renal biopsy in a 6-year-old girl with gross hematuria.

on-site pathologist, who evaluates the adequacy of the specimen. FNA may be performed using 22-gauge to 25-gauge needles, which, if adequate, may obviate a core biopsy. At the end of the procedure, some have advocated the use of Gelfoam slurry or pledgets.[21] At our institution, we typically do not use these techniques for this procedure.

Spleen

In the past, the spleen has been avoided as a target for biopsy, out of fear of bleeding, as well as its proximity to the colon and lung pleura. However, multiple studies have shown splenic biopsy to be a relatively safe procedure.[25–30] Indications for a splenic biopsy include evaluation of a simple cyst, echinococcal cyst, dermoid cyst, hematoma, lymphoma, metastases (melanoma, hepatoma, endometrial carcinoma, gastric tumor), infarct, hemangioma, and hemangiosarcoma.[29] As with hepatic and renal biopsy, clotting factors should be brought to within the acceptable range. The procedure begins with taking initial images of the patient's spleen using a curved array, 3.5-MHz to 5-MHz transducer.[27,28] If more than 1 lesion is

present, the most peripheral lesion should be selected for biopsy. In addition, if the lesion is large enough, the periphery of the lesion itself should be targeted to obtain the most cellular material, because the center may be filled with necrotic debris. For lesions that are in a superior location within the spleen or near the diaphragm, an angled approach may necessary. After administration of local anesthetic, a 20-gauge or 22-gauge biopsy needle for FNA or 18-gauge needle for core biopsy is advanced into the lesion under ultrasound guidance.[29,30]

The most serious complication from splenic biopsy is bleeding. On rare occasions, if conservative management fails, splenic artery embolization or splenectomy may be required.[25,29] Other possible complications may arise from puncturing neighboring structures, such as pneumothorax or empyema from puncturing the diaphragm, or bowel perforation.[27,29]

Management of Immediate Complications

One of the most common complications that occur immediately after the procedure is bleeding. The interventional radiologist must be aware

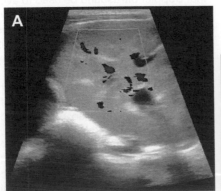

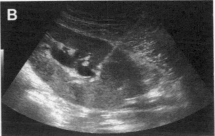

Fig. 4. (A) Use of color Doppler on a renal transplant to locate blood vessels to avoid them. This technique should be performed before passing a needle, as shown in (B).

of bleeding from different sources such as the skin, intercostal location, liver (either contained within the capsule or from the parenchyma, which can result in either a capsular hematoma or hemoperitoneum), or hemobilia. The appropriate measures are taken, such as administering IV fluids and correcting the underlying cause, such as coagulopathy or hypertension. In rare circumstances, the interventional radiologist may need to perform an angiogram and embolize the source of bleeding with either Gelfoam or coils.[15]

The other frequent complication is pain at the puncture site. Typically pain is managed with IV narcotics. The IV route is the quickest onset of action and shortest duration. Thus this is the preferred method in comparsion to oral or intramuscular route. Nonsteroidal antiinflammatory drugs are avoided because they cause an increased risk of bleeding. Continuous pain may require a physical examination and further imaging with either ultrasound or a CT scan.

COMPLICATIONS
Liver

An ultrasound percutaneous liver biopsy is a relatively safe procedure, with minimal complications. The overall risk is 0.2% to 0.3%.[31] The most frequent complications are bleeding and pain in the region. Bleeding at the site is a common occurrence, particularly for patients with underlying liver disease or coagulopathy. Kim and colleagues[32] describe a sign called the patent track sign on Doppler sonography as an early detection for post-biopsy bleeding. In addition, close attention must be paid to patients with hypervascular neoplasms or hemangiomas.[33] If patients have an underlying coagulopathy, vitamin K or fresh frozen plasma is administered.

The less common and major complications are pneumothorax, infection, and seeding within the needle track. Pneumothorax is rare occurrence and is only concerning in patients with lesions close to the pleura. The incidents are reported as only 0.5%.[17] Therefore, the patient's oxygen saturation should be closely observed. If there is further clinical suspicion, a chest radiograph is recommended for further evaluation.

Another rare, but significant, occurrence is seeding within the needle track of biopsy in patients with hepatocellular carcinoma. This complication is particularly concerning in patients who are potential recipients of liver transplant. The incidence ranges from 0.6% to 5.1%. However, Maturen and colleagues[19] have reported that the use of a coaxial system reduces the rate to 0%.

Kidney

A renal biopsy is considered a relatively safe procedure, with an overall mortality of 0.031%. The complications are bleeding, pseudoaneurysm formation, arteriovenous fistula, infection, injury to adjacent organs, and tumor seeding. Bleeding can occur within the collecting system, which causes hematuria, or there may be subcapsular bleeding, results in a subcapsular hematoma, or perinephric bleeding, which evolves into a retroperitoneal hematoma. Therefore, serial hematocrit levels and cross-sectional imaging are necessary for follow-up and further evaluation.[16] A pseudoaneurysm or an arteriovenous fistula can be assessed with color duplex Doppler. An arteriogram with Gelfoam or coil embolization may be required for further management. The incidence of tumor seeding of renal mass is rare, with only 7 cases reported in the literature.[9]

SUMMARY

Ultrasound-guided biopsy of the liver, kidney, and spleen has become integrated into the mainstream of medical management to obtain an adequate specimen. This modality has been proved to be cost-effective, safe, and to avoid any ionizing radiation. Therefore, it should be the primary modality used to obtain a diagnosis.

REFERENCES

1. Hergesell O, Felten H, Andrassy K, et al. Safety of ultrasound-guided percutaneous renal biopsy–retrospective analysis of 1090 consecutive cases. Nephrol Dial Transplant 1998;13(4):975–7.
2. Maya ID, Allon M. Percutaneous renal biopsy: outpatient observation without hospitalization is safe. Semin Dial 2009;22(4):458–61.
3. Zerbino DD. Biopsy: its history, current and future outlook. Lik Sprava 1994;(3–4):1–9 [in Russian].
4. Grant A, Neuberger J. Guidelines on the use of liver biopsy in clinical practice. British Society of Gastroenterology. Gut 1999;45(Suppl 4):IV1–11.
5. Alwall N. Aspiration biopsy of the kidney, including i.a. a report of a case of amyloidosis diagnosed through aspiration biopsy of the kidney in 1944 and investigated at an autopsy in 1950. Acta Med Scand 1952;143(6):430–5.
6. Iversen P, Brun C. Aspiration biopsy of the kidney. 1951. J Am Soc Nephrol 1997;8(11):1778–87 [discussion: 1778–86].
7. Kark RM, Muehrcke RC. Biopsy of kidney in prone position. Lancet 1954;266(6821):1047–9.
8. Goldberg B, Pollack MH, Kellerman, et al. Ultrasonic Localization for Renal Biopsy. Radiology 1975;115:167–70.

9. Uppot RN, Harisinghani MG, Gervais DA. Imaging-guided percutaneous renal biopsy: rationale and approach. AJR Am J Roentgenol 2010;194(6):1443–9.

10. Fuiano G, Mazza G, Comi N, et al. Current indications for renal biopsy: a questionnaire-based survey. Am J Kidney Dis 2000;35(3):448–57.

11. Maturen KE, Nghiem HV, Caoili EM, et al. Renal mass core biopsy: accuracy and impact on clinical management. AJR Am J Roentgenol 2007;188(2): 563–70.

12. Guyatt GH, Akl EA, Crowther M, et al, American College of Chest Physicians Antithrombotic Therapy and Prevention of Thrombosis Panel. Executive summary: antithrombotic therapy and prevention of thrombosis, 9th ed: American College of Chest Physicians evidence-based clinical practice guidelines. Chest 2012;141(Suppl 2):7S–47S.

13. Martin ML, Lennox PH. Sedation and analgesia in the interventional radiology department. J Vasc Interv Radiol 2003;14(9 Pt 1):1119–28.

14. Siskin G. Outpatient care of the interventional radiology patient. Semin Intervent Radiol 2006;23(4): 337–45.

15. Hatsiopoulou O, Cohen RI, Lang EV. Postprocedure pain management of interventional radiology patients. J Vasc Interv Radiol 2003;14(11):1373–85.

16. Dogra V, Saad W. Ultrasound guided procedures. New York: Thieme Medical; 2010. p. 3–34.

17. Shankar S, van Sonnenberg E, Silverman SG, et al. Interventional radiology procedures in the liver. biopsy, drainage, and ablation. Clin Liver Dis 2002; 6(1):91–118.

18. Van Ha TG. Liver biopsy in liver transplant recipients. Semin Intervent Radiol 2004;21(4):271–4.

19. Maturen KE, Nghiem HV, Marrero JA, et al. Lack of tumor seeding of hepatocellular carcinoma after percutaneous needle biopsy using coaxial cutting needle technique. AJR Am J Roentgenol 2006; 187(5):1184–7.

20. Hatfield MK, Beres RA, Sane SS, et al. Percutaneous imaging-guided solid organ core needle biopsy: coaxial versus noncoaxial method. AJR Am J Roentgenol 2008;190(2):413–7.

21. Zins M, Vilgrain V, Gayno S, et al. US-guided percutaneous liver biopsy with plugging of the needle track: a prospective study in 72 high-risk patients. Radiology 1992;184(3):841–3.

22. Sahni VA, Silverman SG. Biopsy of renal masses: when and why. Cancer Imaging 2009;9:44–55.

23. Sharma KV, Venkatesan AM, Swerdlow D, et al. Image-guided adrenal and renal biopsy. Tech Vasc Interv Radiol 2010;13(2):100–9.

24. Ahmad I. Biopsy of the transplanted kidney. Semin Intervent Radiol 2004;21(4):275–81.

25. Gomez-Rubio M, Lopez-Cano A, Rendon P, et al. Safety and diagnostic accuracy of percutaneous ultrasound-guided biopsy of the spleen: a multicenter study. J Clin Ultrasound 2009;37(8):445–50.

26. Kang M, Kalra N, Gulati M, et al. Image guided percutaneous splenic interventions. Eur J Radiol 2007;64(1):140–6.

27. Keogan MT, Freed KS, Paulson EK, et al. Imaging-guided percutaneous biopsy of focal splenic lesions: update on safety and effectiveness. AJR Am J Roentgenol 1999;172(4):933–7.

28. Lucey BC, Boland GW, Maher MM, et al. Percutaneous nonvascular splenic intervention: a 10-year review. AJR Am J Roentgenol 2002;179(6):1591–6.

29. Venkataramu NK, Gupta S, Sood BP, et al. Ultrasound guided fine needle aspiration biopsy of splenic lesions. Br J Radiol 1999;72(862):953–6.

30. Solbiati L, Bossi MC, Bellotti E, et al. Focal lesions in the spleen: sonographic patterns and guided biopsy. AJR Am J Roentgenol 1983;140(1):59–65.

31. Piccinino F, Sagnelli E, Pasquale G, et al. Complications following percutaneous liver biopsy. A multicentre retrospective study on 68,276 biopsies. J Hepatol 1986;2(2):165–73.

32. Kim KW, Kim MJ, Kim HC, et al. Value of "patent track" sign on Doppler sonography after percutaneous liver biopsy in detection of postbiopsy bleeding: a prospective study in 352 patients. AJR Am J Roentgenol 2007;189(1):109–16.

33. Heilo A, Stenwig AE. Liver hemangioma: US-guided 18-gauge core-needle biopsy. Radiology 1997; 204(3):719–22.

Ultrasound-Guided Biopsies of Superficial Structures (Thyroid and Lymph Nodes)

Edward J. Mathes, PA-C[a,b]

KEYWORDS

- Fine-needle aspiration • Thyroid nodules • Lymph nodes • Superficial lesions • Ultrasonography
- Biopsy

KEY POINTS

- All thyroid and many soft-tissue lesions are readily biopsied using ultrasound guidance.
- Using a styletted needle and sterile normal saline as an acoustic coupling agent markedly reduces sample artifact.
- Smaller needles (25-gauge) typically provide a better sample, with less blood artifact than larger (22-gauge or larger) needles.
- Reviewing all samples at the time of procedure allows for immediate operator technique adjustments to improve specimen quality.
- Working closely with the Pathology and Cytology departments will reduce sampling error and improve patient and referrer satisfaction.

 Videos of ultrasound-guided biopsy techniques accompany this article

INTRODUCTION

Over the past several decades, ultrasound-guided core and fine-needle aspiration (FNA) biopsy of thyroid and other soft-tissue lesions has proved to be a cost-effective, sensitive method for obtaining diagnostic tissue samples. Ultrasonography allows one to visualize in real time the smaller, nonpalpable lesions in areas that are otherwise inaccessible. Critical, nearby structures can be seen and avoided, and there is no exposure to ionizing radiation for the operator and patient.

FNA sensitivity is high, with reported accuracy for thyroid nodules ranging from 57% to 95%, with an experienced operator.[1,2] Structures most amenable to ultrasound core biopsy or fine-needle aspiration include breast cysts and masses, thyroid nodules, solid soft-tissue lesions, lymph nodes, and ganglion. Other cystic lesions may be accessed and aspirated using ultrasound.

This article focuses on the essentials of thyroid lesion biopsy, patient comfort, specimen handling, and tips to improve technique and maximize results. The techniques presented are easily applied to nonthyroid soft-tissue lesions.

FINE-NEEDLE ASPIRATION

FNA, needle aspiration biopsy (NAB), fine-needle aspiration cytology (FNAC), and fine-needle aspiration biopsy (FNAB) are all terms used to describe

Conflict of interest: None.
Funding: Departmental source.
a Division of Vascular and Interventional Radiology, Department of Imaging Sciences, Strong Memorial Hospital, 601 Elmwood Avenue, Rochester, NY 14642, USA; b Physician Assistant Program, Rochester Institute of Technology, Rochester, NY, USA
E-mail address: Edward_Mathes@urmc.rochester.edu

Ultrasound Clin 8 (2013) 155–163
http://dx.doi.org/10.1016/j.cult.2012.12.011
1556-858X/13/$ – see front matter © 2013 Elsevier Inc. All rights reserved.

the use of a thin-walled, fine-gauge (usually a 22–25-gauge) needle that is inserted into a lesion to sample cells to be examined under a microscope. This technique may be performed by palpation, whereby the operator can feel a superficial nodule or mass; or by using imaging guidance for smaller or deeper lesions. There are 2 generally accepted techniques: capillary action, by agitating the needle up and down within the lesion thereby driving cells up the hollow needle shaft, or by applying suction to the needle, usually with a syringe. There are several commercial devices to facilitate suction, such as the Tao Aspirator. Both techniques are acceptable but, in the author's experience, capillary action sampling is less traumatic and less prone to sampling errors caused by bloody smears. Lesion sampling via FNA is also less traumatic than a core or open surgical biopsy. Complications are few, often limited to soreness at the puncture site and minor bruising.

Box 1
Risk factors for thyroid cancer

- Male gender
- Nodules occurring before the age of 30 or after the age of 60 years
- History of head and neck radiation
- Family history of thyroid cancer
- Rapid growth of a nodule
- Compressive symptoms (hoarseness, dysphasia, cough)
- Firm, hard nodules that may be fixed to surrounding tissue
- Regional adenopathy
- Nodules larger than 1 cm, indicating malignancy

CORE BIOPSY

A core biopsy is a percutaneous technique whereby a special biopsy device that removes a piece, or core, of tissue is used. There are multiple manufacturers of these devices (Cook, Temno, Bard), which range in size from 12-gauge to 20-gauge. These devices are used in cases where cellular architecture is important to secure a diagnosis, as in most lymphomas, liver disease, and some gastrointestinal and lung cancers. Technique often includes using imaging to direct a larger-diameter coaxial needle percutaneously until the tip abuts the tumor, then passing the biopsy device through the coaxial needle to obtain the sample.

THYROID

Palpable thyroid nodules are fairly common in the adult and pediatric populations, having an incidence of 4% to 7% in an iodine-sufficient population.[3,4] Nodules found incidentally via nontarget imaging (chest computed tomography or cervical magnetic resonance imaging), suggest a prevalence of 19% to 67%.[5,6] The true incidence remains obscure. In a 1955 Mayo Clinic study, thyroid nodules were found in 50.5% of 821 consecutive autopsies of patients with clinically normal thyroid glands.[7] Thyroid nodules are 4 times more common in women than in men[6] and occur more often in people who live in geographic areas with iodine deficiency. Thyroid carcinoma occurs in roughly 5% to 10% of palpable nodules.[1] Risk factors for thyroid cancer are listed in **Box 1**. Ionizing radiation exposure to the neck increases

the risk of the development of thyroid nodules at a rate of 2% annually. In the hands of experienced operators, FNA can be diagnostic for several lesions such as papillary carcinoma, anaplastic carcinoma, medullary carcinoma, follicular neoplasm, Hashimoto thyroiditis, colloid goiter, and large-cell lymphoma.

The initial medical evaluation will differentiate those patients requiring FNA from those that may be monitored over time. The primary objective is to differentiate malignant from benign disease.

Most patients presenting for FNA will have undergone extensive medical evaluation. In 2009, the American Thyroid Association published management guidelines for patients with thyroid nodules.[6] Medical history and physical examination, laboratory evaluation, and FNA of the nodule(s) are all important components of the evaluation. Ultrasonography of the thyroid is the most sensitive way of detecting nodules as small as 2 mm (**Fig. 1**). Ultrasonographic features that raise suspicion of cancer include hypoechoic nodules, nodules with microcalcifications, and irregular nodules. However, given the sensitivity and cost-effectiveness of FNA, many clinicians refer for FNA early in the evaluation process.

PATIENT PREPARATION

Patient preparation is paramount. A recent medical history, general and directed physical examination, and minimal laboratory studies are needed. These procedures should identify those patients at risk for complication, the most significant being bleeding at the biopsy site. If the patient is on anticoagulants, medication should be stopped after

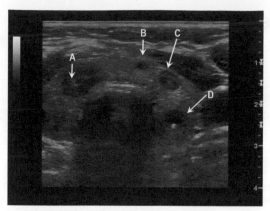

Fig. 1. Example of a multinodular goiter examined using normal saline as the acoustic coupler rather than gel. Arrows A, C, and D are examples of cystic/solid nodules. Nodule A contains microcalcifications. Arrow B indicates a small cyst.

Box 2
The Bethesda System for reporting thyroid cytopathology: recommended diagnostic categories

I. Nondiagnostic or Unsatisfactory

Cyst fluid only

Virtually acellular specimen

Other (obscuring blood, clotting artifact, and so forth)

II. Benign

Consistent with a benign follicular nodule (includes adenomatoid nodule, colloid nodule, and so forth)

Consistent with lymphocytic (Hashimoto) thyroiditis in the proper clinical context

Consistent with granulomatous (subacute) thyroiditis

Other

III. Atypia of Undetermined Significance or Follicular Lesion of Undetermined Significance

IV. Follicular Neoplasm or Suspicious for a Follicular Neoplasm

Specify if Hürthle cell (oncocytic) type

V. Suspicious for Malignancy

Suspicious for papillary carcinoma

Suspicious for medullary carcinoma

Suspicious for metastatic carcinoma

Suspicious for lymphoma

Other

VI. Malignant

Papillary thyroid carcinoma

Poorly differentiated carcinoma

Medullary thyroid carcinoma

Undifferentiated (anaplastic) carcinoma

Squamous cell carcinoma

Carcinoma with mixed features (specify)

Metastatic carcinoma

Non-Hodgkin lymphoma

Other

consultation with the referring physician. The International Normalized Ratio should be less than 1.5 and the platelet count greater than 50,000 to minimize the risk of bleeding. Aspirin and nonsteroidal anti-inflammatory medications have minimal impact on bleeding and can be withheld or not at the operator's discretion. Most superficial FNA and biopsy procedures will not require conscious sedation. However, in selected patients, an oral dose of a short-acting benzodiazepine such as midazolam can be used. The recommendation is nothing by mouth except medications with a sip of water for a minimum of 6 hours before the procedure.

FNA TECHNIQUE

The goal of FNA is to obtain an adequate sample for diagnosis. Until recently there has been little consistency in reporting results, often leading to confusion in interpreting such results.[8] The author's institution uses the Bethesda System for Reporting Thyroid Cytopathology (Box 2, Figs. 2–4, Table 1).[9]

Correct interpretation requires adequate sampling. The author has the benefit of immediate bedside cytologic examination of FNA material to determine adequacy using Romanowski, Dip-Quick or Wrights stain. Additional slides are also wet fixed in 95% ethyl alcohol for Papanicolaou staining. In general, a minimum of 6 clusters containing 10 or more follicular cells are required to call a sample "adequate." Any remaining material in the FNA needle and syringe should be rinsed in normal saline and examined by the cytopathologist.

Cysts and colloid nodules will, because of their primarily liquid nature, yield scant material. The presence of abundant colloid is almost always a sign of a benign lesion. Colloid nodules and cysts should be aspirated and the aspirate sent to cytology (Fig. 5). If there is a solid component to the cystic lesion, it should be sampled after aspiration to rule out a cystic papillary cancer. Simple cysts will yield numerous macrophages, whereas

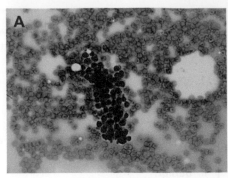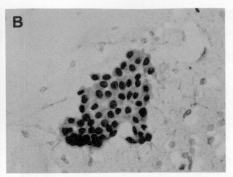

Fig. 2. (*A, B*) Thyroid, left bed, ultrasound-guided fine-needle aspiration. Malignant tumor cells derived from papillary thyroid carcinoma are present. (*A*) 6× magnification Wrights stain. (*B*) 10× magnification papanicolaou stain.

hemorrhagic cysts will contain hemosiderin. Thyroiditis (Hashimoto, autoimmune, or chronic lymphocytic thyroiditis) is characterized by the presence of large numbers of lymphocytes and macrophages. Hypercellular smears with scant or no colloid favors a diagnosis of neoplasm.

METHOD

Obtaining an adequate tissue sample for cytologic evaluation is not a simple task. Administration of local anesthetic, visualization of the nodule, and tracking the needle tip require a deft hand and dexterity. Sample contamination from ultrasound gel and/or blood should be minimized, as they can hinder examination (**Fig. 6**).

Once the nodule is identified by ultrasonography, the skin is marked. Lidocaine 1% is administered subdermally using a 30-gauge needle and 1- to 3-mL syringe. The lidocaine is not injected directly into skin ("raising a skin weal"), but subcutaneously, and allowed to back diffuse into skin. Depending on the nodule location, the thyroid capsule may also be injected. Thyroid FNA is performed using a 22- to 25-gauge styletted, 4.5-cm length spinal needle.

Using a linear ultrasound probe, the needle is visualized and tracked through subcutaneous tissue, the thyroid capsule, and into the central portion of the nodule (**Fig. 7**). One may use an aspiration technique, using a syringe and gentle aspiration while agitating the needle tip in the nodule, or a capillary technique whereby the needle is aggressively agitated within the nodule, driving cells up the hollow shaft. No syringe or suction is used with the capillary technique. The needle itself is rotated between the thumb and finger while agitating to change the cutting angle of the needle bevel. The needle is removed once material appears in the hub. Cystic thyroid lesions should be evacuated first using a larger (20–22-gauge) needle and syringe (see **Fig. 5**). Once collapsed, the solid component can be sampled.

Immediate cytology examination is used to determine sample adequacy. Bedside examination of the sample provides immediate feedback, allowing you to correlate technique with results, adjusting as necessary to improve sample collection.

Sample contamination is a concern. The thyroid is rich in capillary blood vessels. Sampling using the aspiration technique typically contains

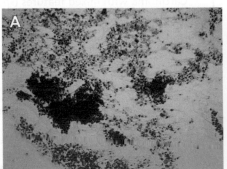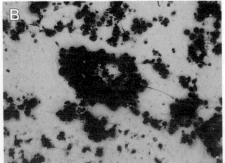

Fig. 3. (*A, B*) Low- and high-power stained images: Malignant tumor cells derived from poorly differentiated carcinoma. (*A*) 4× magnification Wrights stain. (*B*) 10× magnification papanicolaou stain.

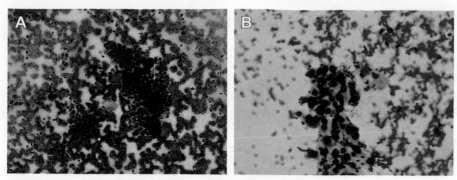

Fig. 4. (*A, B*) The aspirate is highly cellular, with oncocytic groups and numerous blood vessels. Marked nuclear crowding with pseudoinclusions, grooves, and papillary-like fragments are noted. A papillary thyroid carcinoma, oncocytic variant, is in the differential. (*A*) 10× magnification Wrights stain. (*B*) 10× magnification papanicolaou stain.

Table 1
The bethesda system for reporting thyroid cytopathology: implied risk of malignancy and recommended clinical management

Diagnostic Category	Risk of Malignancy (%)	Usual Management[a]
Nondiagnostic or unsatisfactory	1–4	Repeat FNA with ultrasound guidance
Benign	0–3	Clinical follow-up
Atypia of undetermined significance or follicular lesion of undetermined significance	~5–15[b]	Repeat FNA
Follicular neoplasm or suspicious for a follicular neoplasm	15–30	Surgical lobectomy
Suspicious for malignancy	60–75	Near-total thyroidectomy or Surgical lobectomy[c]
Malignant	97–99	Near-total thyroidectomy[c]

Abbreviation: FNA, fine-needle aspiration.
[a] Actual management may depend on other factors (eg, clinical, sonographic) besides the FNA interpretation.
[b] Estimate extrapolated from histopathologic data from patients with "repeated atypicals."
[c] In the case of "Suspicious for metastatic tumor" or a "Malignant" interpretation indicating metastatic tumor rather than a primary thyroid malignancy, surgery may not be indicated.
Data from Cibas ES, Ali SA. The Bethesda system for reporting thyroid cytopathology Am J Clin Pathol 2009;132: 658–65; with permission.

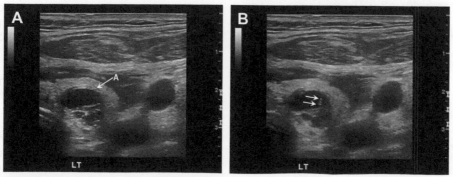

Fig. 5. (*A*) Primarily cystic nodule (*arrow*). (*B*) A 20–22-gauge needle positioned in the liquid component for aspiration (*double arrow*).

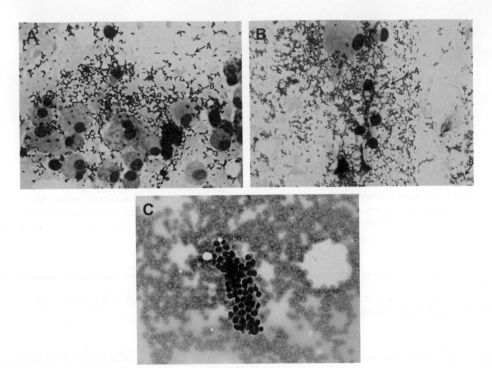

Fig. 6. (*A, B*) High-power quik-diff stain demonstrates ultrasound gel crystallization (*arrows A and B*). (*C*) High-power quik-diff stain without gel contamination (*arrows A and B*).

significant amounts of blood. Blood artifact can be minimized by using a smaller needle, using the capillary technique, and limiting the procedure to less than 5 seconds.[10] Gel contamination is eliminated by using a styletted needle (removing the stylet once the needle tip is in the nodule) and using sterile normal saline as the ultrasound acoustic coupling agent. In our experience, image quality is not degraded when using normal saline or sterile water instead of gel (see **Fig. 6**).

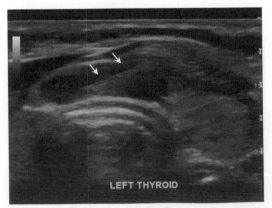

Fig. 7. A 25-gauge needle within a large anterior cervical lymph node (*arrows*).

CORE BIOPSY OF THYROID

Several studies comparing core needle biopsy with FNA of thyroid nodules have been published.[11–13] Core biopsy sampling is a safe and effective alternative to FNA of thyroid nodules. The author reserves core sampling for those patients in whom previous FNA is nondiagnostic, there is inadequate specimen, or when lymphoma is suspected. Biopsy is performed using a technique similar to that of FNA. An 18- or 20-gauge single-action spring-activated core biopsy needle with a 1.1-cm throw (Cook Quick-Core, Inrad SelectCore, Temno Evolution, others) is directed into the nodule under ultrasound guidance, being careful not to overpenetrate the thyroid into extracapsular tissue (**Fig. 8**). Tissue is placed in formalin and transported to pathology for processing.

Core biopsy has the advantage of providing a larger volume of tissue than FNA, aiding in diagnosis. The reported sensitivity, specificity, and accuracy for FNA ranges from 90% to 93%, 60% to 70%, and 80% to 85%, respectively. For core-needle biopsy, reported results are 92% to 96%, 75% to 80%, and 85% to 90%, respectively. Core-needle biopsy is safe while carrying a higher incidence of bleeding and patient discomfort than FNA.[11–13]

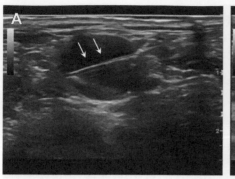
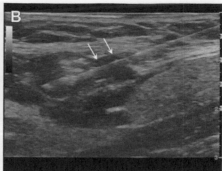

Fig. 8. (*A*) Enlarged lymph node being biopsied using a 20-gauge core device (*arrows*). (*B*) Core biopsy needle within a nodule (*arrows*).

Box 3
Common soft-tissue masses

Benign Soft-Tissue Masses
- Infection (bacterial, viral, fungal, other)
- Lipoma
- Angiolipoma
- Fibroma
- Benign fibrous histiocytoma
- Neurofibroma
- Schwannoma
- Neurilemmoma
- Hemangioma
- Giant-cell tumor of tendon sheath
- Myxoma

Malignant Soft-Tissue Masses
- Carcinoma (primary and metastatic)
- Melanoma
- Myeloma
- Dermatofibrosarcoma protuberans
- Lipoma
- Hemangioma
- Lymphangioma
- Peripheral nerve sheath tumor
    - Schwannoma
    - Neurofibroma
- Malignant fibrous histiocytoma
- Liposarcoma
- Leiomyosarcoma
- Epithelioid sarcoma
- Nodular fasciitis
- Fibromatosis

Several other soft-tissue masses are amenable to ultrasound-directed FNA and core biopsy. **Box 3** lists the more common benign and malignant soft-tissue masses, lipoma and enlarged cervical/supra-clavicular/axillary lymph nodes being the most common (**Figs. 9** and **10**).

The biopsy technique for these lesions is similar to that described for thyroid. In many cases, core-needle biopsy is the technique of choice given the differences in cellular architecture among tumors. More tissue is better. We often use FNA of these masses with immediate cytologic evaluation is used to differentiate viable from necrotic tissue, allowing targeting of an area with a greater probability of diagnosis. The lesion is then biopsied using a 16- to 20-gauge single-action, spring-loaded, adjustable-length biopsy gun (eg, Bard Monopty, BioPince Full Core, Temno, Cook). Size selected is based on lesion size, location, and presumed diagnosis. Most specimens are collected, placed on a normal saline-soaked Telfa pad, then immersed in formalin before transport to pathology. If lymphoma is suspected, the more tissue made available for analysis the better. Tissue is obtained

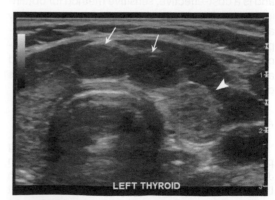

Fig. 9. Enlarged cervical lymph nodes (*arrows*) to be sampled using fine-needle aspiration.

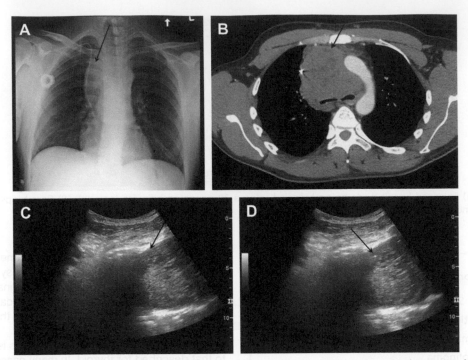

Fig. 10. (*A*) Chest radiograph demonstrating large mediastinal mass (*arrow*). (*B*) Computed tomography scan of mediastinal mass (*arrow*). (*C*) Ultrasonographic appearance of mediastinal mass (*arrow*). (*D*) A 25-gauge needle tip in lesion (*arrow*).

using a larger, 14- to 16-gauge core biopsy device. Tissue is placed fresh on a saline-soaked Telfa pad and immediately transported to pathology in a dry sterile container. Additional cells are obtained using FNA at time of core biopsy and submitted for flow cytometry.

Complications, including bleeding, infection, and discomfort at the biopsy site, are rare.

SUMMARY

Ultrasound-directed FNA and core biopsy of thyroid and other soft-tissue nodules carries minimal risk and is a cost-effective, sensitive method for obtaining tissue samples for diagnosis. Ultrasonography allows one to visualize in real time the smaller, non-palpable lesions in areas that are otherwise inaccessible. FNA sensitivity is high, with a reported accuracy ranging from 60% to 95% in the hands of an experienced operator.[1,2]

ACKNOWLEDGMENTS

The author would like to thank the following people for their contributions to this article: Ellen J. Giampoli, MD, Director, fine-needle aspiration biopsy service, Associate Professor, Department of Pathology and Laboratory Medicine, University of Rochester Medical Center, School of Medicine and Dentistry; and Donna K. Russell, MEd, CT(ASCP)HT, Supervisor of Cytopathology Residency, University of Rochester Medical Center, School of Medicine and Dentistry.

VIDEOS

Videos related to this article can be found online at http://dx.doi.org/10.1016/j.cult.2012.12.011.

REFERENCES

1. Gharib H, Goellner JR. Fine-needle aspiration biopsy of thyroid: an appraisal. Ann Intern Med 1993;118: 282–9.
2. Oertel YC. Fine-needle aspiration of the thyroid: techniques and terminology. Endocrinol Metab Clin North Am 2007;36:737–51, vi–vii.
3. Vander JB, Gaston EA, Dawber TR. The significance of nontoxic thyroid nodules: final report of a 15 year study of the incidence of thyroid malignancy. Ann Intern Med 1968;69:537–40.
4. Mazzaferri EL. Thyroid cancer in thyroid nodules: finding a needle in the haystack. Am J Med 1992; 93:359–62.
5. Tan GH, Gharib H. Thyroid incidentalomas: management approaches to nonpalpable nodules discovered incidentally on thyroid imaging. Ann Intern Med 1997; 126:226–31.

6. Cooper DS, Doherty GM. American Thyroid Association management guidelines for patients with thyroid nodules and differentiated thyroid cancer. Thyroid 2009;19(11):1167–214.

7. Brander A, Viikinkoski P, Nickels J, et al. Thyroid gland: US screening in a random adult population. Radiology 1991;181:683–7.

8. Mortensen JD, Woolner LB, Bennett WA. Gross and microscopic findings in clinically normal thyroid glands. J Clin Endocrinol Metab 1955;15:1270–80.

9. Cibas ES, Ali SA. The Bethesda system for reporting thyroid cytopathology. Am J Clin Pathol 2009;132: 658–65.

10. Nguyen GK, Ginsberg J, Crockford PM. Fine-needle aspiration biopsy cytology of the thyroid. Its value and limitations in the diagnosis and management of solitary thyroid nodules. Pathol Annu 1991;25: 63–91.

11. Quinn SF, Nelson HA, Demlow TA. Thyroid biopsies: fine-needle aspiration biopsy versus spring-activated core biopsy needle in 102 patients. J Vasc Interv Radiol 1994;5(4):619–23.

12. Harvey JN, Parker D, De P, et al. Sonographically guided core biopsy in the assessment of thyroid nodules. J Clin Ultrasound 2005;33(2):57–62.

13. Samir AE, Vij A, Seale MK, et al. Ultrasound-guided percutaneous thyroid nodule core biopsy: clinical utility in patients with prior nondiagnostic fine-needle aspirate. Thyroid 2012;22(5):461–7 [Epub 2012 Feb 3].

Ultrasound-Guided Biliary Intervention
Can Radiation Risk Be Reduced?

Shirley Chan, MD[a],*, Devang Butani, MD[b]

KEYWORDS

- Cholecystostomy • Percutaneous transhepatic cholangiogram • Real-time dosimetry • Biliary stent

KEY POINTS

- Enhance the noninterventional radiologist's knowledge about how biliary procedures are performed from a technical standpoint.
- Educate all readers on how radiation exposure to both operator and patient can be decreased or in some cases, even eliminated.

INTRODUCTION

This article reviews common biliary procedures, such as cholecystostomy tube and percutaneous transhepatic cholangiogram (PTC) with biliary stent placement, while focusing on radiation exposure reduction through the use of ultrasound, fluoroscopy, and real-time dosimetry.

DISCUSSION
Cholecystostomy

The current gold standard for acute cholecystitis is a cholecystectomy. The few patients who have serious contraindications for general anesthesia or are not medically stable for the operating room with American Society of Anesthesiologists 3 or 4 classification, however, require cholecystostomy tube placement. The current medical community considers cholecystostomy tube placement as a minimally invasive, safe, and temporizing measure to relieve the acute obstruction until a patient can be cleared for surgery.[1] Recent studies show that this procedure significantly reduces morbidity and

mortality.[2,3] Widely accepted indications for this procedure include acalculus and calcular cholecystitis, bile leak, decompression of malignant obstruction, and conjunction with fluoroscopically and endoscopic-guided gallstone removal.[4]

The first step in cholecystostomy tube placement is determining a suitable needle trajectory. Some interventional radiologists prefer one that transverses a small portion of the inferior edge of the right liver lobe (**Figs. 1** and **2**) to minimize the risk of bile leaks and subsequent bile peritonitis, a painful clinical complication. Using this approach, however, commits patients to having a drainage catheter for 4 to 6 weeks while the tract matures. If the drain is removed before this time frame, there is a higher risk of hepatic bleeding from the immature tract. For this reason, some interventionalists favor a direct puncture.

A direct puncture approach eliminates the risk of hepatic bleeding, and the cholecystostomy tube can be removed earlier. Unfortunately, the risk of bile leak is higher with this approach. There is also literature that suggests that gallbladder aspiration

a Department of Imaging Sciences, University of Rochester Medical Center, 601 Elmwood Avenue, Box 648, Rochester, NY 14624, USA; b Division of Interventional Radiology, Department of Imaging Sciences, University of Rochester Medical Center, 601 Elmwood Avenue, Box 648, Rochester, NY 14624, USA
* Corresponding author.
E-mail address: shirley_chan@urmc.rochester.edu

Ultrasound Clin 8 (2013) 165–170
http://dx.doi.org/10.1016/j.cult.2012.12.005
1556-858X/13/$ – see front matter © 2013 Elsevier Inc. All rights reserved.

ultrasound.theclinics.com

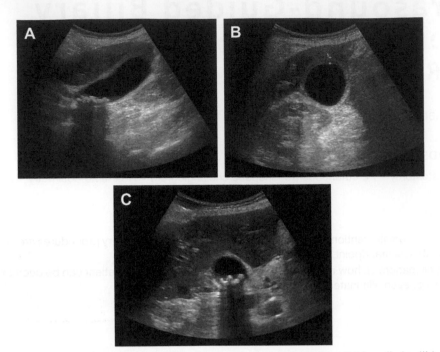

Fig. 1. (A–C) Right upper quadrant ultrasound showing acute cholecystitis with a thick-walled gallbladder (5 mm) containing small stones and sludge.

without a drain is sufficient to stabilize patients emergently.[5] A semielective cholecystectomy can be performed subsequently once patients become more stable.

Advances in ultrasound technology, including dynamic 2-D ultrasound mounted on steering guidance system (ATL Philips, Bothell, Washington, USA), provides better visualization of the needle tip with a controlled trajectory.[4] The ultrasound transducer is set to low frequency with typical ranges of 2 MHz to 5 MHz for deep organ visualization. The gallbladder is approached anteriolaterally via transhepatic (see **Fig. 2**) or anteriorly via transperitoneal routes.

Once the needle trajectory is determined, a probe with a guide can be used to place a coaxial needle into the gallbladder. If the procedure is performed under ultrasound at a patient's bedside, bile can be aspirated to confirm positioning. A wire is passed through the needle, which can also be viewed with ultrasound. The tract is then dilated, and the drain is placed over the wire. Ultrasound visualization of the drainage catheter within the gallbladder can be used for documentation (see **Fig. 2**D). Overall, this entire procedure can be performed under ultrasound guidance.

Ultrasound offers the advantages of real-time and continuous visualization, low cost, portability, vascular and biliary anatomy analysis, and, more

importantly, lack of ionizing radiation. Thus, ultrasound is the first-line choice for imaging guidance, at least for initial access, with CT guidance as a secondary choice in the event of poor sonographic visualization of the gallbladder. Common reasons for CT guidance are contracted gallbladder, collapsed gallbladder wall due to rupture, shrunken gallbladder size from chronic inflammation with thickened wall and viscous intraluminal contents, extreme patient obesity, and recent oral or caffeine intake.[6] The latter can be easily remedied by ensuring nothing-by-mouth status of patients before the procedure.

Percutaneous Transhepatic Cholangiogram and Biliary Drains

Interventional radiology has much to offer for both diagnosis and management of acute and chronic biliary disease. The majority of procedures involve imaging and decompression of biliary ductal disease via PTC, with or without biliary drain placement. In patients with biliary obstruction and impedance of biliary flow above the insertion of the cystic duct, percutaneous drainage is preferred to endoscopic biliary drainage due to the specific target-guided decompressive capabilities of this procedure. Using a percutaneous approach, the clinician can plan for biliary stent placement in the focally obstructed bile duct

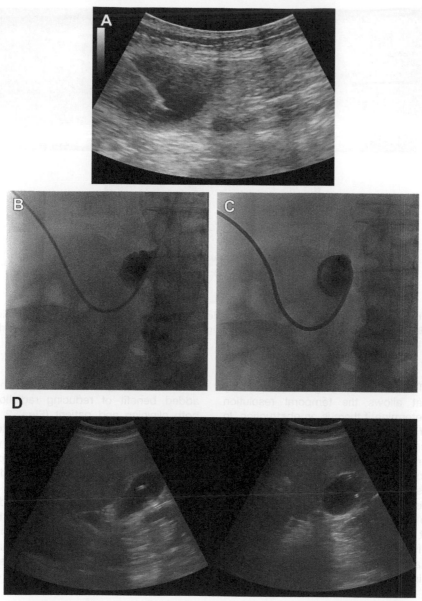

Fig. 2. (*A*) Intraprocedural ultrasound showing the needle tip within a distended gallbladder. (*B*) Catheter and guide wire were passed into the gallbladder via a transhepatic approach and trace amount of contrast was injected. (*C*) Pigtail catheter was placed in the gallbladder. (*D*) Ultrasound images confirming pigtail catheter within the lumen of the gallbladder.

branch and/or drainage of the more functionally preserved liver segments. PTC involves placing a small-caliber needle into a bile duct with subsequent injection of contrast to opacify and image the bilary tree. If an obstruction is encountered, the obstructed segments can be decompressed by placement of a biliary drain.

One of the unfavorable aspects of a PTC is the significant amount of radiation exposure, especially to the operator hands and while accessing

the left biliary tree. The majority of the exposure occurs during the initial attempts at accessing the biliary tree with a Chiba needle. Ultrasound can be used to guide the placement of the Chiba needle into a dilated biliary radical, thus eliminating the largest portion of radiation exposure.

In liver transplant patients with elevated liver enzymes, PTC is the procedure of choice because bile ducts in a transplant patient do not tend to be dilated even in the presence of an obstructive

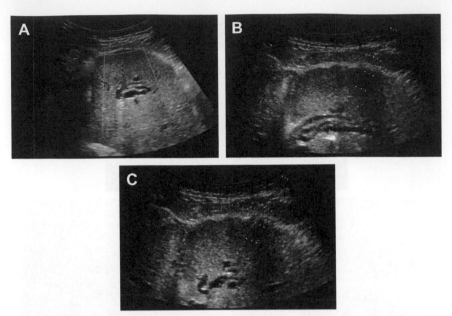

Fig. 3. (*A*) Left hepatic lobe ultrasound with color Doppler showing the targeted portal triad containing a dilated biliary duct. (*B*). Grayscale images with guidance showing the needle trajectory toward the biliary duct. (*C*) Echogenic needle tip in the dilated bile duct.

pathology. Thus, a cholangiogram is the only modality that allows the temporal resolution needed to determine if there is an obstruction. In the setting of adequate drainage, hepatic dysfunction in this subset of patients can then be attributed to transplant rejection or other organic causes. Unfortunately, ultrasound may be not as useful in these patients as opposed to those who have ductal dilation.

Access to the biliary system can be obtained from the left with a subcostal approach or from the right with a midaxillary intercostal approach. Either side has distinct advantages and disadvantages. The initial portion of a left PTC is often performed using ultrasound guidance with the added benefit of reducing radiation doses to both clinician and patient (**Figs. 3** and **4**). The transducer is set on color Doppler to distinguish biliary from vascular flow and to visualize the targeted peripheral biliary radical to puncture.

A right PTC is usually performed under fluoroscopic guidance. The intercostal trajectory of the needle makes ultrasound guidance nearly impossible. Extra measures must be taken by the clinician and ancillary staff to reduce radiation doses. Intrahepatic ductal dilatation enhances visualization of the biliary tree and targeted biliary radical, thereby reducing the

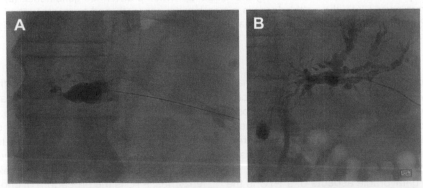

Fig. 4. Contrast injection at early (*A*) and later phases (*B*) confirms needle tip placement and outlines the dilated left biliary tree with high-grade stenosis of the central left bile duct. Note the normal caliber of the common bile duct.

A B

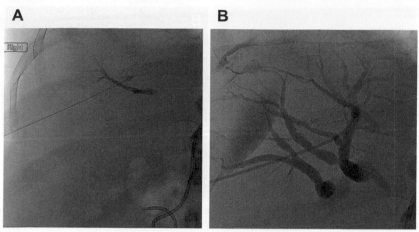

Fig. 5. (*A*) Right PTC under fluoroscopic guidance shows needle insertion in a peripheral right bile duct. The patient has a previously placed left internal external biliary stent. (*B*) Insertion of catheter with contrast outlining the right biliary tree.

number of attempts needed to obtain access (**Fig. 5**).

Methods to reduce radiation doses, as recommended by the American College of Radiology imaging gently campaign, are applicable to biliary procedures. These include wearing properly fitting lead aprons, thyroid shields, and leaded eyewear; positioning and collimating while fluoroscopy is off; excluding radiation to sensitive parts of the body, such as the eyes, breast, thyroid, and reproductive organs; using table shields and overhanging lead shields; using extension tubing or power injector when injecting by hand; adjusting acquisition parameters to accommodate the lowest dose for patient size; slower frame rate; and minimization of magnification (**Fig. 6**).[7]

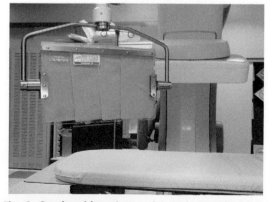

Fig. 6. Overhead hanging and upright standing lead shields are designed to reduce ionizing radiation to the upper body and lower body, respectively.

Real-time Dosimetry

Poor operator technique is an occult and often longstanding contributor to unnecessary ionizing radiation doses to clinicians and ancillary staff. Some of these habits can be resolved by proper training and education or better supervision. Cumulative ionizing radiation exposure, however, has a long observer period before manifestation of clinical symptoms, usually monitored retrospectively by dosimeters quarterly or monthly in most institutions, and is undetectable by the senses, making it difficult for clinicians to receive real-time feedback to quickly adjust their work pattern.

The recent development of a real-time dosimeter can resolve this issue. The University of Rochester Interventional Radiology Division is a test site for 1 of 2 commercially available real-time dosimetry systems. The DoseAware Personal Dose Meter System (Philips Healthcare, Andover, MA, USA) is a solid-state electronic dosimeter with a high-capacity memory that detects scattered x-ray photons and spontaneously displays individualized readings as color-coded bar graphs on a nearby base station screen via wireless technology (**Fig. 7**). Thus, it provides clinicians and ancillary staff with real-time feedback to recognize intraprocedural work patterns that contribute to high radiation doses. In response, interventionalists can quickly develop adaptive measures to improve personal safety.[8]

Preliminary reports from the authors' institution have shown significant reduction in overexposure rates. Internal audits that track as-low-as-reasonably-achievable letters show 88% and 78% reduction in respective level 1 and level 2

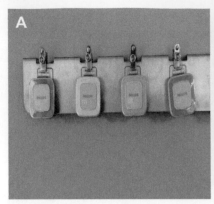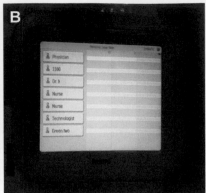

Fig. 7. (*A*) Individualized Philips Healthcare DoseAware dosimetry badges are displayed on the wall of the angiography suite. (*B*) When worn, the dosimetry badge transmits the real-time radiation dose (mSv) that is displayed on a monitor.

overexposure rates over the course of the initial 3 months trial period.

SUMMARY

Many methods exist to reduce cumulative radiation dose in interventional radiology biliary procedures. A combination of all strategies, including using proper protective equipment, using proper technique, selection of low radiation dose imaging guidance, and simplifying the complexity of cases, will effectively minimize the sequelae of radiation exposure and maximize patient and clinician safety.

REFERENCES

1. Cherng N, Witkowski ET, Sneider EB, et al. Use of cholecystostomy tubes in the management of patients with primary diagnosis of acute cholecystitis. J Am Coll Surg 2012;214(2):196–201.
2. Morse BC, Smith JB, Lawdahl RB, et al. Management of acute cholecystitis in critically ill patients: contemporary role for cholecystostomy and subsequent cholecystectomy. Am Surg 2010; 76(7):708–12.
3. Chung YH, Choi ER, Kim KM, et al. Can percutaneous cholecystostomy be a definitive management for acute acalculous cholecystitis? J Clin Gastroenterol 2012;46(3):216–9.
4. Ginat D, Saad WE. Cholecystostomy and transcholecystic biliary access. Tech Vasc Interv Radiol 2008; 11(1):2–13.
5. Ito K, Fujita N, Noda Y, et al. Percutaneous cholecystostomy versus gallbladder aspiration for acute cholecystitis: a prospective randomized controlled trial. Am J Roentgenol 2004;183(1):193–6.
6. Hanbidge AE, Buckler PM, O'Malley ME, et al. From the RSNA refresher courses: imaging evaluation for acute pain in the right upper quadrant. Radiographics 2004;24(4):1117–35.
7. Hernanz-Schulman M, Goske MJ, Bercha IH, et al. Pause and pulse: ten steps that help manage radiation dose during pediatric fluoroscopy. Am J Roentgenol 2011;197(2):475–81.
8. Sanchez R, Vano E, Fernandez JM, et al. Staff radiation doses in a real-time display inside the angiography room. Cardiovasc Intervent Radiol 2010;33(6):1210–4.

Tumor Ablation
Ultrasound Versus CT

Joseph Reis, MD*, Devang Butani, MD

KEYWORDS

• Cryoablation • Radiofrequency • Ablation • Ultrasound • CT

KEY POINTS

• Explain the limitations and advantages of cryoablation and radiofrequency ablation (RFA).
• Understand the physics of sonoelastography, contrast-enhanced ultrasound, RFA, and cryoablation.
• Decide when to use ultrasound or computed tomography for image-guided ablation.

INTRODUCTION

Cancer is the second most common cause of mortality in the United States, leading to more than 500,000 deaths annually.[1] Surgery, radiation therapy, and chemotherapy have represented the mainstay of treatment for neoplasms before the development of interventional oncology. The advent of interventional oncology has broadened the scope of multimodality cancer treatment.

Hepatic tumors were early targets of percutaneous and intraoperative ablation, given their ease of direct access. Percutaneous ethanol and radiofrequency ablation (RFA) for hepatocellular carcinoma (HCC) treatment began in the late 1980s and early 1990s.[2–5] HCC has the second lowest 5-year survival rate among cancer subtypes and has significantly increased in incidence over the past 20 years with a 12.3% increase among males in the United States from 2001 to 2007.[6–8] Ablation is currently used to treat hepatocellular carcinoma in nonoperative candidates, to serve as a bridge to transplantation, and to serve as a palliative measure. Percutaneous ablation of metastatic disease to the liver, such as colorectal cancer, is also increasing. Less commonly treated metastatic tumors include breast cancer and neuroendocrine tumors (relief of hormone-related symptoms).[9] Developing interventional oncology

therapies and improvements in traditional techniques have contributed to the 14.9% increase in 5-year survival rates for localized hepatocellular carcinoma from 2001 to 2007.[6]

Renal cell carcinoma (RCC) detection is also increasing, partially because of incidental discovery on computed tomography (CT).[10,11] Approximately 69% of RCC is discovered incidentally.[12,13] The small size and low grade of these tumors at the time of detection has prompted interest in nephron-sparing ablation procedures.[14,15] RFA and cryoablation are the most commonly used procedures.[16,17] These techniques have demonstrated promising results in long-term follow-up studies.[18,19]

Percutaneous ablation requires imaging guidance. Options include ultrasound (US), CT, and magnetic resonance imaging (MRI). Imaging serves 5 key roles: planning, targeting, monitoring, controlling, and assessing treatment response.[20] Each modality has unique advantages. US is cost-effective and provides real-time imaging, whereas CT provides an excellent field of view and real-time capabilities.[21] MRI provides excellent resolution, but is limited by cost and procedure time.

This review compares US and CT guidance for RFA and cryoablation of renal and hepatic neoplasms, as these are the most common ablation procedures.

Disclosures: The authors of this article have nothing to disclose.
Department of Imaging Sciences, University of Rochester Medical Center, 601 Elmwood Avenue, Box 648, Rochester, NY 14642-8648, USA
* Corresponding author.
E-mail address: Joseph_Reis@urmc.rochester.edu

Ultrasound Clin 8 (2013) 171–183
http://dx.doi.org/10.1016/j.cult.2012.12.006

OVERVIEW OF RFA AND CRYOABLATION

Tumor ablation was defined as "the direct application of chemical or thermal therapies to a specific focal tumor (or tumors) in an attempt to achieve eradication or substantial tumor destruction" by the International Working Group on Image-Guided Tumor Ablation in 2005, dividing the technique into chemical and thermal categories.[20] Irreversible electroporation has since emerged as an alternate method of ablation. Thermal ablation remains the most popular method of choice, specifically RFA and cryoablation.[16]

Ablation is most commonly used for the treatment of tumors within the kidney and liver. Indications for RFA and cryoablation overlap, although there are differences.

Early-stage isolated HCC is optimally treated with surgical resection in appropriate candidates.[22] Unfortunately, less than 15% of HCC meets these criteria in patients with cirrhosis who are poor surgical candidates.[23] Ablation is advocated for treatment of a single HCC focus of 5 cm or smaller or 3 areas of HCC in the liver each 3 cm or smaller; however, recent studies suggest that surgical therapy 5-year survival rates may be superior to RFA percutaneous ablation survival rates in tumors 3 cm or larger.[23] Metastatic tumor ablation work has primarily focused on colorectal carcinoma metastases isolated to the liver, although treatment of other metastases is growing. Contraindications to treatment of hepatic metastases include tumor size of 4 cm or larger in maximal diameter and overwhelming tumor burden in the liver.[24]

Conservative treatment is commonly advocated for renal masses smaller than 1 cm, given that 44% of these masses are benign and 25% of masses smaller than 3 cm are benign.[25] Indications for intervention include large masses, rapid growth (>3 mm/y), progressive enlargement on serial examinations, or prophylactic removal to ease patient concerns. Lesion size is also a limiting factor; upper limits for tumor sizes are 4 to 5 cm in longest dimension.[26,27] Ablation may be performed, however, in patients with larger tumors who are nonoperative candidates. Additional specific indications for renal ablation include nephron-sparing therapy for renal tumors in patients with baseline renal insufficiency, single kidneys, transplant kidneys and hereditary syndromes predisposing to renal tumors. Nononcologic indications for RFA include control of chronic hematuria and postbiopsy bleeding.[28]

Both intraoperative and percutaneous ablation techniques may be used, although there is an increasing trend toward percutaneous procedures, given the relative decrease in hospitalization time.

Preprocedural evaluation includes a consultation with the patient explaining risks and benefits of the ablation, evaluation of coagulopathy, review of medication allergies, consultation with a hepatologist or nephrologist to establish baseline organ function, and imaging review. Imaging review is essential before the procedure to determine lesion accessibility and screen for potential complications.

The optimal treatment scenario for a renal tumor is an exophytic solid lesion located posteriorly away from vessels and adjacent organs or bowel. Intraparenchymal lesions and central lesions pose a greater risk of damage to the renal hilum and collecting system, although the complication rate in cryoablation is lower than that of RFA.[29] Exophytic tumors are usually protected by a rim of surrounding retroperitoneal fat that can serve as an insulator from surrounding structures during RFA. Solid tumors respond best to RFA.[29] Cystic tumors may require repeat ablations to treat each of their solid components. These difficulties have led some to suggest that cystic tumors should be treated only when they have a greater than 50% solid component.

US VERSUS CT IN SCREENING AND TUMOR CHARACTERIZATION

US is a cost-effective treatment modality in screening high-risk patients for HCC and in patients with hematuria or unexplained renal failure. Individual lesions also may be characterized with acoustically enhancing microbubbles or sonoelastography. However, once a lesion is discovered, CT or MRI is commonly obtained to screen for additional occult parenchymal tumors and metastatic disease. Ultrasound has an advantage of quickly identifying and characterizing a single hepatic or renal lesion, but may fail to detect additional smaller foci of involvement.

Although b-mode US is cost-effective, subtle tumors can often be missed because of their isoechoic imaging characteristics or because of distortion of surrounding normal anatomy, such as in patients with cirrhosis. Uses of b-mode US include screening for occult tumors during intraoperative ablation. Occasionally, tumors may not be visible on a triphasic preprocedural CT scan but are visible on intraoperative US before ablation.[30] This has not been demonstrated with percutaneous US, likely because of suboptimal visualization of hepatic tumors relating to poor acoustic transmission, low probe frequency, and overlying artifacts.

Some institutions currently use contrast-enhanced US (CEUS) to screen for tumors in high-risk patients. Intravenous contrast agents consist of gas containing bubbles with diameters of approximately 40 μm that enhance acoustic reflection in flowing blood.[31] Early in contrast US development, acoustic enhancement agents were taken up by the liver over a period of 5 minutes followed by a high-intensity US sweep across the liver that caused the bubbles to burst.[32] The final image demonstrated focal hypoechoic areas representing tumor involvement. This method had limited application to interventional procedures and allowed only single-phase cine imaging. Subsequently, a pulse inversion imaging technique was developed in which alternated positive and negative pulses were applied to the microbubbles at optimized mechanical indices, allowing vascular imaging of tumors in multiple phases similar to CT and MRI multiphase contrast imaging.[32] This imaging technique allows the characterization of lesions and procedural localization of tumors in a number of organs, including the liver, kidney, and prostate.[33] US combined with color and power Doppler images can further aid in depicting areas of parenchymal hypervascularity from a focal lesion.

Sonoelastography is an alternate method of focused tissue characterization. Elastography is a measure of axial tissue displacement resulting from static waves generated by an external source. Displacement may be created using quasistatic compression waves or vibration.[34] Quasistatic compression produces strain forces on tissue that can be measured on Doppler US.[34] Vibration waves generate a shear wave as the tissue returns to its original orientation.[34] Velocities of generated shear waves are directly proportional to the tissue elastic modulus.[35] Differences in local tissue strain can then be fused with sonographic images to generate contrast between normal tissue and tumors. Hepatic tumors have increased stiffness relative to surrounding parenchyma, allowing for contrast distinction. Sonoelastography can also be used to differentiate between certain tumor histologies. For example, cholangiocarcinoma is significantly stiffer than hepatocellular carcinoma and metastases to the liver, whereas lymphoma has a low stiffness.[36]

Both CEUS and sonoelastography have limitations. CEUS cannot assess metastatic disease as well as CT or MRI and may miss tumors near the diaphragm because of pulmonary and motion artifacts. Limitations of sonoelastography are low spatial resolution, probe sliding, vibration-generated probe movement, respiratory motion, and patient motion. Controlled breathing and the use of ablation probes as sources of vibration or compression have improved some of the limitations.

ABLATION PROCEDURE BASICS

The procedure begins with patient positioning in the supine, prone, decubitus, or oblique orientations. US, CT, or MRI is obtained and the area of entry is sterilized and draped. The patient is anesthetized with conscious sedation, such as intravenous fentanyl and midazolam. Once the patient is comfortable and in position, repeat images are obtained to determine the exact location of entry.[28] Any of the 3 imaging modalities may be used to guide probe placement, but US has the advantage of real-time guidance.

Distancing the ablation probes from nontarget organs and vital structures is imperative before beginning the procedure. Hydrodissection can be used to create a fluid plane between target organs and adjacent vital structures, such as the colon, stomach, and gallbladder surrounding the liver or the adrenal gland or ilioinguinal and iliofemoral nerves surrounding the kidney. Vital structures, such as the renal collection system, gallbladder, and bile ducts, can be avoided by choosing an appropriate probe angle and ablation method.

US VERSUS CT IN PROBE GUIDANCE AND HYDRODISSECTION

US is the modality of choice for hydrodissection given the real-time monitoring and nonradiation. The US probe is angled over the site of insertion and a 22-G Chiba needle is carefully advanced along the path with slow injection of approximately 50 to 100 mL of D5W and eventual creation of a hydroplane between adjacent vital structures and the organ of interest (**Fig. 1**).

Artificial ascites have a greater benefit compared with an artificial pleural effusion, which is associated with pneumonia and respiratory dysfunction. Ascites can be protective against surrounding injury for most hepatic lesions; however, do not prevent diaphragmatic injury during hepatic dome ablations.[37]

Following hydrodissection, US is used to guide applicator probe placement (**Fig. 2**). The goal of placement is to center probes within the target lesions and reposition them as needed during the procedure to achieve adequate treatment margins. Residual tumor is difficult to detect on b-mode US, resulting in repeat ablation sessions, increased health care cost, and risk to the patient.

Mistargeting of tumor is another difficulty associated with b-mode US. Mistargeting refers to ablation of a pseudolesion without any ablation of the actual tumor. Improper electrode placement, poor sonographic windows, cirrhotic liver morphology, and poor intrinsic conspicuity of the target lesion

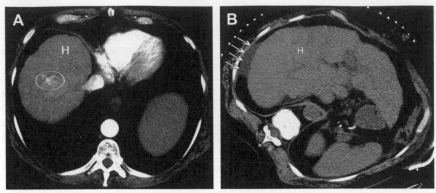

Fig. 1. Hydrodissection before RF ablation. Arterial-phase contrast CT (*A*) demonstrates a focal enhancing lesion (*circle*) at the dome of the liver (H). (*B*) D5W solution is then injected (*arrows*) into the perihepatic fat lateral adjacent to the right hepatic lobe (H) and confirmed with noncontrast CT.

on US lead to suboptimal treatment.[38] Improper probe placement is related to both inexperience and a poor sonographic window. The sonographic window can be obscured by overlying bowel gas, lung shadowing, and rib shadows. Contrasted CT may be required in these cases to accurately guide placement of the probes. Cirrhotic livers and inconspicuous lesions may similarly require CT. Clear

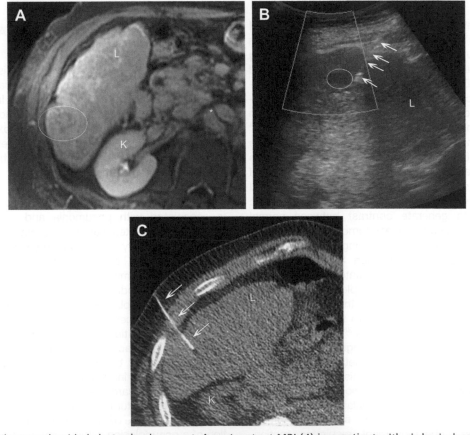

Fig. 2. Ultrasound-guided electrode placement. A postcontrast MRI (*A*) in a patient with cirrhosis demonstrates a lesion with mixed portal venous phase enhancement (*circle*) in the right hepatic lobe (L). (*B*) US with color Doppler is used to identify the hypoechoic lesion (*circle*) to guide electrode placement (*arrows*). (*C*) Noncontrast CT confirms the position of the probe (*arrows*) in the liver (L). *, incidental aortic dissection; K, kidney.

Causes of Mistargeting

- Improper electrode placement
- Poor sonographic window
- Cirrhotic liver morphology
- Poor conspicuity of target lesion

localization of the lesion on planning US, with or without contrast and elastography, helps avoid these complications.

RFA

RFA is the application of heat transmitted from electromagnetic radio waves to induce cellular death through coagulative necrosis in human tissue. Heat is generated from water molecules. Water molecule dipole moments align with the direction of applied radio waves. Alternating current changes the direction of dipole moments, causing water molecules to vibrate rapidly and transfer kinetic energy to the tissues.[39] Cell death results from the breakdown of proteins with temperature-sensitive moieties that denature above 50°C.[5,40] Once tissue temperatures increase above 105°C, cellular vaporization and charring occur.[39]

Radio waves are transmitted through a monopolar internally cooled electrode, bipolar electrodes, saline perfusion electrodes, or a group of expandable thin metal tine electrodes that fan out from the tip.[39] Separate probes may be spaced at approximately 1 cm for large tumors to increase the zone of ablation.[39] Single electrodes ablate in a spherical configuration, whereas multiple electrodes create a dumbbell-shaped zone of coverage (**Fig. 3**C). Energy deposition from the probes is localized to the area of interest by creation of a closed loop circuit using 2 anode grounding pads placed on the patient's posterior thigh.

The electrodes generally have coverage of 2 to 5 cm, depending on the configuration of the electrodes.[39] Smaller zones of ablation are desired for tumors adjacent to vital structures, but the optimal ablation zone should produce 1-cm tumor-free margins.[41]

Temperatures of 50 to 100°C are maintained for 10 to 30 minutes with serial monitoring of progress on imaging.[41] Only 4 to 6 minutes of heating is required to kill cells at these temperatures in vitro, but longer heating times are usually required in vivo because of nonideal conduction efficiencies from the probe to the tissue.[41] Thermocouples measure the temperature at the electrode tips and adjust the power needed to maintain probe temperature accordingly.

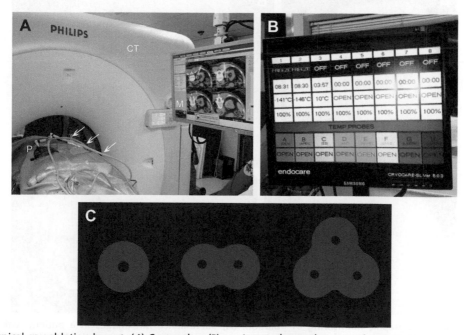

Fig. 3. Typical cryoablation layout. (*A*) Cryoprobes (P) are inserted over the area of percutaneous access that has been prepped and draped under sterile conditions. Heavy cryoablation cords (*arrows*) must be properly placed to avoid torquing of the probes. (*B*) Temperatures of the electrodes are continuously monitored with thermocouples. (*C*) Each of the probes placed (*black dots*) produce somewhat rounded ablation zones (*red*) that overlap when placed near each other. M, monitor.

Typical power requirements range from 150 to 250 W in liver.[41] Initial trials performed on renal tumors demonstrated that much less power was required for ablation, on the order of 50 W.[41] Greater heat loads result in excessive tissue damage and increased the risk of renal infarction because of the lack of a dual blood supply from the kidney and small organ size compared with the liver. As tissues necroses, the power necessary to heat the probes decreases with a roll of the tissue impedance.

A cool-down mode is then used, followed by a track ablation mode during which the electrodes are retracted and the electrode tracts are coagulated, thereby maintaining a tissue temperature above 70°C.[41]

The heat sink effect discussed previously has a more significant impact on renal tumors than hepatic tumors because of the increased blood flow to the kidneys and relatively high vascularity. Indicators of inadequate tissue ablation depend on the type of equipment used and may include persistent low temperatures during the ablation phase of the procedure, rapid temperature decline during cooling, a post-RFA temperature maximum of less than 70°C, lack of generator pulsations, and decreased impedance.[28]

US VERSUS CT IN MONITORING RFA

RFA ablation monitoring may be performed with US, CT, or MRI. US has the advantage of real-time imaging, low cost, and availability, but incompletely demonstrates the ablation zone. Sonographic images demonstrate an enlarging echogenic ablation zone near the tip of the probe originally thought to represent coagulation necrosis, but now known to correspond with echogenic interfaces from tiny gas bubbles (**Fig. 4**).[42] Distinguishing ablated tissue from viable tumor is therefore difficult given the mixed echogenicity of tumors and architectural

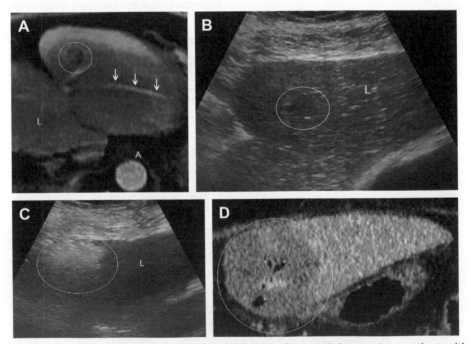

Fig. 4. B-mode sonographic monitoring of ablation. (*A*) Surveillance MR images in a patient with cirrhosis demonstrate a focal lesion (*circle*) with portal venous washout in the left lobe of the liver (L). (*B*) Gray-scale US is used to localize the lesion (*circle*). (*C*) Following ablation, the ablated region is hyperechoic and obscured by dirty shadowing from microbubbles (*circle*). (*D*) Postablation contrast CT demonstrates a hypoechoic zone of ablation (*circle*) with pneumobilia and air (*asterisk*) that is larger than the hyperechoic region visible on US. A, aorta; arrows, left portal veins.

distortion produced by the ablation.[42] The probe tip also becomes difficult to visualize for repositioning.[43] Power and color Doppler modes have not been shown to improve detection of residual tumor.[44] This limitation has been addressed with CEUS and sonoelastography.

CEUS relies on the concept that ablated tissue will not enhance, because the vessels in that tissue are coagulated. Viable tumor demonstrates residual vascularity, which is evidenced by enhancement or blood flow detected in the ablation (**Fig. 5**). Contrast enhances the sensitivity of flow detection on both color and power Doppler.[45] Power harmonic Doppler is more sensitive than color Doppler imaging in detecting backscatter from intravascular microbubbles and is therefore more commonly used.[46,47]

CEUS is currently slightly less sensitive than CT for detection of residual tumor, but has the benefit of detecting blood flow solely within vessels rather than detecting enhancement in both the intravascular and extravascular spaces.[48]

Therefore, CEUS may be used as a screening tool to detect viable tumor following ablation with subsequent CT imaging if the scan is negative (**Fig. 6**). This provides an affordable method to detect residual tumor requiring immediate reintervention.

Sonelastography is useful for measuring the zone and borders of ablated tissues both in vitro and in vivo (**Fig. 7**). Elastography tends to slightly underestimate the 3-dimensional volume of hepatic tissue ablated when correlated with pathologic specimens.[49] Similar underestimation of the treated volume following ablation has also been demonstrated for renal lesions.[50] Determining the preprocedural tumor volume helps to ensure adequate lesion coverage during ablation.

As tumoral tissue is ablated, protein denaturation occurs and the elastic modulus of the tissue is elevated. Furthermore, elastic modulus changes as temperatures increase in necrosed tissue, allowing for a quantitative assessment of thermal dose deposition.[51] Limitations occur with

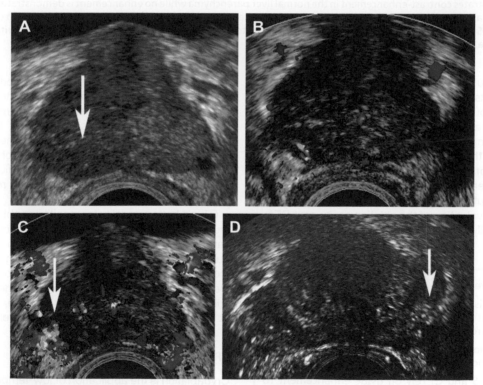

Fig. 5. CEUS in the prostate. (A) Gray-scale images of the prostate demonstrate an ill-defined hypoechoic area in the peripheral zone of the prostate near the capsule (*arrow*). (B) Color Doppler images demonstrate flow within this area similar to the rest of the gland. (C) CEUS with color Doppler better localizes the tumor, which is extremely hypervascular. (D) Gray-scale CEUS in a different patient clearly delineates a hyperechoic focus in the peripheral zone concerning for adenocarcinoma. Definity contrast (1 vial in 50-mL normal saline administered intravenously over 10 minutes) was used. (*Courtesy of* Dr Ethan Halpern at the Jefferson Prostate Diagnostic Center of Thomas Jefferson University as part of an NIH-funded protocol to investigate contrast-enhanced imaging of the prostate.)

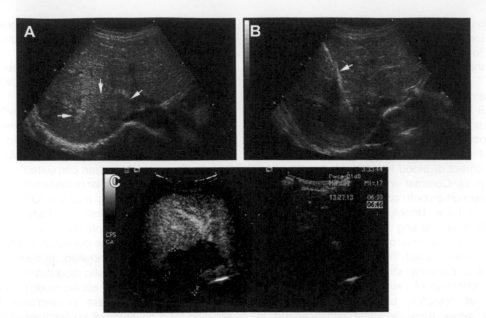

Fig. 6. CEUS imaging used to confirm the effectiveness of RFA therapy. Pre-RFA conventional US imaging (*A*) demonstrates a poorly defined area (*arrows*) in this patient with known liver metastases. (*B*) The RFA needle (*arrow*) was inserted into the tumor area under US guidance. Contrast-enhanced US performed immediately post-RFA (*C*) demonstrates contrast-enhancement in the normal liver parenchyma while no enhancement is demonstrated in the treated area (Note: This is a dual display that demonstrates phase-inversion harmonic US on the left and a conventional US image on the right). (*Courtesy of* Daniel A. Merton, BS, RDMS, Thomas Jefferson University Hospital, Philadelphia, PA.)

microbubble formation during the ablation. Large amounts of microbubbles cause increased posterior acoustic shadowing that limits visualization of the distal ablation boundary. This limitation can be overcome by waiting 30 to 60 minutes before evaluating the ablation zone with sonoelastography. Most of the microbubbles clear at 30 minutes and nearly all of the microbubbles clear at 60 minutes.[52]

CT evaluation of the ablation cavity post RFA is optimally performed with contrast. Multiple contrast-enhanced CT scans may be performed before, during, and following ablation to more accurately monitor the extent of tissue necrosis by using smaller amounts of contrast (50-mL increments). Rim enhancement around the cavity is commonly seen in the portal venous phase of scans in the first 24 hours following ablation, and wanes over time.[53] Optimal detection of residual tumor is arterial phase imaging.[53]

CT is a better modality for monitoring ablation of multiple overlapping tumors. Coagulative changes can impede US localization of additional tumor foci during the procedure.[54] CT also allows for frequent monitoring of ablated tissue during the procedure. Elastography and CEUS can be performed only a limited number of times during ablation, usually at the beginning and end of the procedure.

RFA Pearls and Pitfalls

- US is difficult for overlapping zones of ablation secondary to artifact from coagulative necrosis
- Sonoelastography slightly underestimates tumor volume
- CEUS and CT rely on tissue enhancement to detect residual tumor
- Sonoelastography and contrast-enhanced US are generally performed 60 minutes after the procedure
- CT allows more frequent monitoring of ablated tissue during the procedure

---

CRYOABLATION

Cryoablation is the application of low-temperature inert gases to cellular tissues, inducing cell death. Water crystalizes to form ice when rapidly cooled, which disrupts the selective permeability of cell membranes. Damage to intracellular membranes can also activate caspases and trigger apoptosis.[55] Indirect mechanisms of cellular death include dehydration and ischemia. Ice crystal

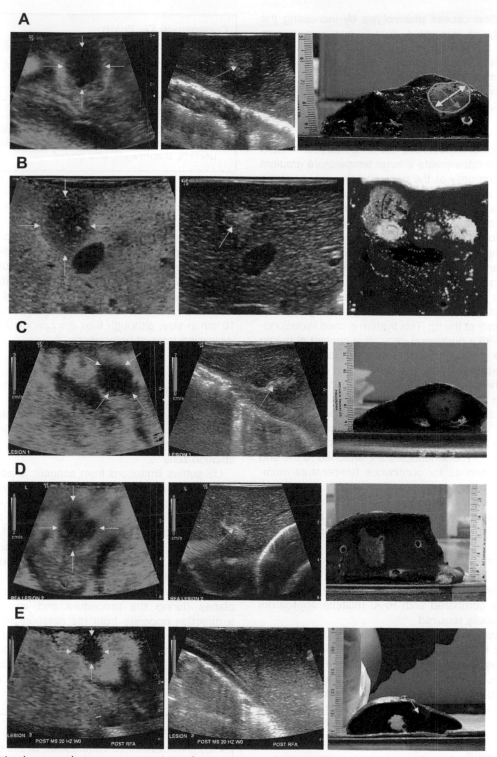

Fig. 7. In vivo sonoelastograms, co-registered sonograms, and gross pathology photographs of RFA lesions. The bright ink on pathology photographs are markers used for later 3-dimensional reconstruction. (*A–E*) The ablation zone is hypoechoic on sonoelastograms with hyperechoic regions on co-registered images (*arrows*) and a clear delineation of the ablation boundaries. Note that liver boundaries induce artifacts on sonoelastograms (*C*) and (*D*). RFA lesions as small as 0.2 cm³ are successfully detected (*E, arrows*). (*From* Zhang M, Castaneda B, Christensen J, et al. Real-time sonoelastography of hepatic thermal lesions in a swine model. Med Phys 2008;35:4132–41; with permission.)

formation causes plasmolysis by increasing the tonicity of interstitial fluid.[55] Ischemia occurs when ice formation damages endothelial membranes, activates an inflammatory response, and induces thrombosis.[55]

Optimal ice crystal formation occurs below −25°C, whereas cellular death occurs below −40°C.[55] Variables affecting cell death include the rates of heating and cooling, as well as the duration of exposure to low temperatures.[55] Rapid cooling rates create a large temperature gradient between cells at the center and periphery of the ablation zone. Freezing and thawing times affect the ice ball size and extent of ice crystal formation.

Cryoprobes produce low temperatures through the Joule-Thompson effect.[55] Rapid volumetric expansion of a gas lowers the gas pressure. Pressure and temperature are roughly proportional, resulting in a significant temperature drop. Argon gas is passed through a narrow slit in the distal aspect of the probe that opens to a large-volume chamber at the tip. This system is used in conjunction with a peripheral circulating coolant at the tip of the probe to optimize heat exchange between the expanding gas and surrounding cells.[55] Up to 8 individual cryoprobes may be placed in relation to the tumor, depending on the desired temperature distribution through the tissue and tumor size.[56] When 3 or more electrodes are placed within 1 cm proximity they are termed cluster electrodes.[56] Thermocouples are attached to the end of the probes for continuous temperature monitoring during the examination.

Probes should be geometrically oriented so that each probe is within 1 cm of the tumor and no more than 2 cm from another probe.[57] Current probes range in length from 13 to 28 cm with a 0°C isotherm zone of 3.2 × 3.4 cm or 3.1 × 3.6 cm to 4.5 × 6.4 cm or 4.0 × 6.7 cm depending on the vendor.[56] Given the smaller ablation zones per probe compared with RFA, multiple applicators are usually required.

Cryoprobes are initially tested in a bowl of sterile water to ensure adequate ice ball formation. The probes are then positioned in and around the lesion. Cryoprobes are connected to cords containing electric wiring and inert gas tubing (see **Fig. 3**). This tubing can weigh down the probes and proper positioning is required relative to the cords to avoid probe torque during the procedure.[56]

The probes are placed into the lesion and the equipment is placed on stick mode, during which the probes quickly freeze in place to secure their positions.[56] At least 2 individual cooling cycles are run to freeze tissue to −20°C.[56] Each cycle lasts approximately 8 to 12 minutes with 8-minute

---

> *Cryoablation Key Points*
> - *Cycles*: At least 2
> - *Time*: 8–12 minutes per cycle, 8-minute intervals
> - *Probes*: Generally 1–4 depending on tumor size, reports of up to 8
> - *Optimal Lesion Location*: Peripheral/Exophytic away from vessels, biliary structures, ureters, diaphragm, and bowel

---

intervals.[56] The treated area is then thawed over 5 minutes using warm helium gas.[56]

High success rates of cryoablation may be because up to 8 probes may be placed, allowing adequate coverage for small tumors and potential ablation therapies for larger tumors. Cryoablation techniques are often used to treat tumors 4 cm or smaller, but may be used to treat tumors up to 10 cm in size, although they are associated with increasing rates of hemorrhage.[58]

US VERSUS CT IN MONITORING CRYOABLATION

Cryoablation has the advantage of clear visibility on CT and US.[18] The ice ball formed during the thermal ablation demarcates the periphery of the ablation zone.

US suffers limitations from acoustic shadowing at the deep end of the ice ball. The impedance of the frozen tissue formed during ablation is significantly different from the deeper nonablated tissue. Therefore, sound waves reaching the interface of the ablation zone and the nonablated tissue will reflect. This produces shadowing and poor visibility of tissue deep to the ice ball. Methods of addressing this problem include imaging in multiple planes during the procedure and imaging in a direction opposite from the ablation probes if the procedure is performed intraoperatively.[59,60] Ablation is often attempted so that the leading edge of the tumor on US moves from distal to proximal. Subsequent shadowing created as the

---

> *Cryoablation Imaging Pearls and Pitfalls*
> - US provides limited visualization of the distal ice ball secondary to acoustic shadowing
> - Multiplanar imaging and intraoperative ablation can decrease US limitations
> - CT easily depicts the cryoablated tissue, which is hyperdense

ice ball forms will obscure the area of ablation, but not more proximal vital structures.[61]

CT has certain advantages over US in cryoablation, most importantly the clear visualization for the ice ball and cryoablation boundary. The boundary represents the 0°C temperature point of tissues at the margin of the probe. Multiphase examinations with small 50-mL alliquots of contrast allows identification of adjacent blood vessels, but are not as useful in detecting residual tumors. There is often nontumoral contrast enhancement immediately following ablation, making residual tumor detection difficult; however, cell death occurs 3 mm deep to the ablation cavity boundaries. The ice ball size can therefore be compared with the preprocedural tumor size to determine the size of ablation zone necessary to achieve adequate coverage. The tumor margin is less well visualized with US in 3 dimensions and reproducible measurements are more difficult depending on the angle at which the tumor is visualized.

SUMMARY

US and CT are 2 commonly used modalities in image-guided tumor ablation. Each provides distinct advantages to both the clinician and patient. US generates real-time images, is readily available, cost-effective, and radiation free. Conversely, CT provides a global picture of the abdomen with sharp delineation of cryoablated tumor boundaries at the cost of radiation to the patient. Current technological developments in contrasted US and sonoelastography allow for improved detection of residual postablation tumor that rival contrasted CT. Operator comfort and details regarding the type and specifics of individual ablations will likely guide the choice of imaging.

What the Referring Physician Needs to Know

- A planning CT or US is required before the ablation procedure
- CT is generally more advantageous than US in monitoring the distal border of cryoablated tissue
- Contrast enhancement on US or CT is a common sign of residual tumor following ablation
- Sonoelastography or CEUS should always be used for RFA; b-mode US alone is not sufficient

REFERENCES

1. Murphy SL, Xu J, Kochanek KD. Deaths: Preliminary Data from 2012. In: NVSR. 2012. Available at: http://www.cdc.gov/nchs/data/nvsr/nvsr60/nvsr60_04.pdf. Accessed June 16, 2012.
2. Livraghi T, Festi D, Monti F, et al. US-guided percutaneous alcohol injection of small hepatic and abdominal tumors. Radiology 1986;161:309–12.
3. Goldberg SN, Gazelle GS, Dawson SL, et al. Tissue ablation with radiofrequency: effect of probe size, gauge, duration, and temperature on lesion volume. Acad Radiol 1995;2:399–404.
4. McGahan JP, Brock JM, Tesluk H, et al. Hepatic ablation with use of radio-frequency electrocautery in the animal model. J Vasc Interv Radiol 1992;3:291–7.
5. McGahan JP, Browning PD, Brock JM, et al. Hepatic ablation using radiofrequency electrocautery. Invest Radiol 1990;25:267–70.
6. American Cancer Society. Cancer facts & figures 2012. Atlanta (GA): American Cancer Society; 2012.
7. El-Serag HB, Mason AC. Rising incidence of hepatocellular carcinoma in the United States. N Engl J Med 1999;340:745–50.
8. Taylor-Robinson SD, Foster GR, Arora S, et al. Increase in primary liver cancer in the UK 1979–94. Lancet 1997;350:1142–3.
9. Gillams A. Tumor ablation: current role in the liver, kidney, lung and bone. Canc Imag 2008;8:S1–5.
10. Pantuck AJ, Zisman A, Belldegrun AS. The changing natural history of renal cell carcinoma. J Urol 2001;166:1611–23.
11. Chow WH, Devesa SS, Warren JL, et al. Rising incidence of renal cell cancer in the United States. JAMA 1999;281:1628–31.
12. Greenlee RT, Hill-Harmon MB, Murray T, et al. Cancer statistics, 2001. CA Cancer J Clin 2001;51:15–36.
13. Jayson M, Sanders H. Increased incidence of serendipitously discovered renal cell carcinoma. Urology 1998;51:203–5.
14. Luciani LG, Cestari R, Tallarigo C. Incidental renal cell carcinoma—age and stage characterization and clinical implications: study of 1092 patients (1982–1997). Urology 2000;56:58–62.
15. Janzen NK, Kim HL, Figlin RA, et al. Surveillance after radical or nephron sparing surgery for localized renal cell carcinoma and management of recurrent disease. Urol Clin North Am 2003;30:843–52.
16. Gervais DA, McGovern FJ, Wood BJ, et al. Radiofrequency ablation of renal cell carcinoma: early clinical experience. Radiology 2000;217:665–72.
17. Atwell TD, Farrell MA, Leibovich BC, et al. Percutaneous renal cryoablation: experience treating 115 tumors. J Urol 2008;179:2136–41.
18. Gill IS, Remer EM, Hasan WA, et al. Renal cryoablation: outcome at 3 years. J Urol 2005;173:1903–7.

19. Gervais DA, McGovern FJ, Arellano RS, et al. Radio-frequency ablation of renal cell carcinoma: part I, indications, results, and role in patient management over a 6-year period and ablation of 100 tumors. AJR Am J Roentgenol 2005;185:64–71.

20. Goldberg SN, Grassi CJ, Cardella JF, et al. Image-guided tumor ablation: standardization of terminology and reporting criteria. J Vasc Interv Radiol 2005;16:765–78.

21. Maybody M. An overview of image-guided percutaneous ablation of renal tumors. Semin Intervent Radiol 2010;27:261–7.

22. Li L, Zhang J, Liu X, et al. Clinical outcomes of radiofrequency ablation and surgical resection for small hepatocellular carcinoma: a meta-analysis. J Gastroenterol Hepatol 2012;27:51–8.

23. Livraghi T. Guidelines for treatment of liver cancer. Eur J Ultrasound 2001;13:167–76.

24. McCarley JR, Soulen MC. Percutaneous ablation of hepatic tumors. Semin Intervent Radiol 2010;3:255–60.

25. Silverman SG, Israel GM, Herts BR, et al. Management of the incidental renal mass. Radiology 2008; 249:16–31.

26. Miki K, Shimomura T, Yamada H, et al. Percutaneous cryoablation of renal cell carcinoma guided by horizontal open magnetic resonance imaging. Int J Urol 2006;13:880–4.

27. Georgiades CS, Hong K, Bizzell C, et al. Safety and efficacy of CT-guided percutaneous cryoablation for renal cell carcinoma. J Vasc Interv Radiol 2008;9:1302–10.

28. Stone MJ, Venkatesan AM, Locklin J, et al. Radiofrequency ablation of renal tumors. Tech Vasc Interv Radiol 2007;2:132–9.

29. Janzen NK, Perry KT, Han KR, et al. The effects of intentional cryoablation and radio frequency ablation of renal tissue involving the collecting system in a porcine model. J Urol 2005;173:1368–74.

30. Wood TF, Rose DM, Chung M, et al. Radiofrequency ablation of 231 unresectable hepatic tumors: indications, limitations and implications. Ann Surg Oncol 2000;7:593–600.

31. Nielsen MB. Contrast enhanced ultrasound. Eur J Radiol 2004;51(Suppl):S1.

32. Nielson MB, Bang N. Contrast enhanced ultrasound in liver imaging. Eur J Radiol 2004;51(Suppl):S3–8.

33. Dietrich CF. Characterization of focal liver lesions with contrast enhanced ultrasonography. Eur J Radiol 2004;51(Suppl):S9–17.

34. Cho N, Moon WK, Kim HY, et al. Sonoelastographic strain index for differentiation of benign and malignant nonpalpable breast masses. J Ultrasound Med 2010;29:1–7.

35. Garra BS. Imaging and estimation of tissue elasticity by ultrasound. Ultrasound Q 2007;23:255–68.

36. Masuzaki R, Tateishi R, Yoshida H, et al. Assessing liver tumor stiffness by transient elastography. Hepatol Int 2007;1:394–7.

37. Kang TW, Rhim H, Lee MW, et al. Radiofrequency ablation for hepatocellular carcinoma abutting the diaphragm: comparison of effects of thermal protection and therapeutic efficacy. AJR Am J Roentgenol 2011;196:907–13.

38. Lee MW, Lim HK, Kim YJ, et al. Percutaneous sonographically guided radiofrequency ablation of hepatocellular carcinoma: causes of mistargeting and factors affecting the feasibility of a second ablation session. J Ultrasound Med 2011;30:607–15.

39. Hong K, Georgiades C. Radiofrequency ablation: mechanism of action and devices. J Vasc Interv Radiol 2010;8:S179–86.

40. Sanchez H, van Sonnenberg E, D'agostine H, et al. Percutaneous tissue ablation by radiofrequency thermal energy as a preliminary to tumor ablation. Minim Invasive Ther Allied Technol 1993;2:299–305.

41. Lencioni R, Crocetti L. Radiofrequency ablation of liver cancer. Tech Vasc Interv Radiol 2007;10:38–46.

42. D'Ippolito G, Goldberg SN. Radiofrequency ablation of hepatic tumors. Tech Vasc Interv Radiol 2002;5: 141–5.

43. Goldberg SN, Gazelle GS, Solbiati L, et al. Ablation of liver tumors using percutaneous RF therapy. AJR Am J Roentgenol 1998;170:1023–8.

44. Solbiati L, Goldberg SN, Ierace T, et al. Hepatic metastases: percutaneous radio-frequency ablation with cooled-tip electrodes. Radiology 1997;205: 367–73.

45. Kim AY, Choi BI, Kim TK, et al. Hepatocellular carcinoma: power Doppler US with a contrast agent—preliminary results. Radiology 1998;209:135–40.

46. Boehm T, Malich A, Goldberg SN, et al. Radiofrequency ablation of VX2 rabbit tumors: assessment of completeness of treatment by using contrast-enhanced harmonic power Doppler US. Radiology 2002;225:815–21.

47. Schwarz KQ, Chen X, Steinmetz S, et al. Harmonic imaging with levovist. J Am Soc Echocardiogr 1997;10:1–10.

48. Solbiati L, Goldberg SN, Ierace T, et al. Radiofrequency ablation of hepatic metastases: postprocedural assessment with a US microbubble contrast agent—early experience. Radiology 1999;211:643–9.

49. Varghese T, Techavipoo U, Liu W, et al. Elastographic measurement of the area and volume of thermal lesions resulting from radiofrequency ablation: pathologic correlation. AJR Am J Roentgenol 2003;181:701–7.

50. Pareek G, Wilkinson ER, Bharat S, et al. Elastographic measurement of in-vivo radiofrequency ablation lesions of the kidney. J Endourol 2006;20: 959–64.

51. Varghese T, Zagzebski JA, Lee FT Jr. Elastographic imaging of thermal lesions in the liver in vivo following radiofrequency ablation: preliminary results. Ultrasound Med Biol 2002;28:1467–73.

Role of Intravascular Ultrasound in Interventional Radiology

Jessica Lee, MD, Nael Saad, MD*

KEYWORDS

- Intravascular ultrasound (IVUS) • Venous thromboembolism
- Bedside inferior vena cava filter placement • Direct intrahepatic portacaval shunt (DIPS)
- Aortic dissection fenestration

KEY POINTS

- Intravascular ultrasound (IVUS) is a valuable tool and adjunct to conventional angiography in endovascular interventions because it allows visualization of vessel wall anatomy as well as adjacent structures.
- IVUS is used for characterization of venous stenosis in the setting of venous thromboembolism and can aid in the differentiation between acute and chronic thrombus and therefore guide decisions regarding therapy.
- Bedside placement of IVC filters under IVUS guidance can be performed in patients with iodinated contrast allergy, pregnancy, weight exceeding limits of the fluoroscopy table, and patients too critically ill for transport.
- IVUS has been used to guide direct puncture from IVC to the portal vein during direct intrahepatic portocaval shunt (DIPS) creation for the treatment of intractable ascites and variceal bleeding.
- IVUS is used in percutaneous balloon fenestration in type B aortic dissection.

 Videos of IVUS during iliac vein thrombolysis, of an aortic dissection, and post motor vehicle accident accompany this article

INTRODUCTION

Since its development in the early 1970s, intravascular ultrasound (IVUS) technology has undergone several improvements in the form of catheters and imaging platforms.[1] These improvements make IVUS a valuable tool and adjunct to conventional angiography in endovascular interventions. Whereas conventional angiography enables visualization of the caliber and contour of a vessel lumen, IVUS enables accurate visualization of vessel wall anatomy as well as adjacent structures and therefore provides important diagnostic information and clinical utility in endovascular interventions,

especially in the setting of complex anatomy that is unclear on angiography.

IVUS BASICS

IVUS uses a small intravascular probe to create a 360° cross-sectional image orthogonal to the long axis of the vessel. Two types of IVUS systems exist: mechanical IVUS and electronic IVUS. Mechanical IVUS is composed of a rotating transducer at the tip of a flexible, high-torque catheter and achieves a 360° image by mechanical rotation of the catheter. In contrast, electronic IVUS uses a fixed circumferential array of up to 64 transducer

Mallinckrodt Institute of Radiology, 510 South Kingshighway Boulevard, St Louis, MO 63110, USA
* Corresponding author.
E-mail address: saadn@mir.wustl.edu

Ultrasound Clin 8 (2013) 185–189
http://dx.doi.org/10.1016/j.cult.2012.12.007

ultrasound.theclinics.com

elements, each producing an individual image in sequence, resulting in a 360° image.[2]

IVUS probes are commercially available in frequencies ranging from 8 to 50 MHz, with catheter diameters ranging from 3 to 9 F.[2] Lower-frequency probes require larger catheters, but as with conventional ultrasound imaging, lower-frequency probes allow for greater depth of tissue penetration. These probes are typically used in femoropopliteal veins and aortoiliac vessels. Higher-frequency probes allow for narrower catheters and improved spatial resolution, but at the cost of depth of sound wave penetration. Therefore, higher-frequency probes are typically used in smaller vessels, such as femoropopliteal arteries and in the coronary vessels.[2] IVUS images allow visualization of the intimal, medial, and adventitial layers of vessels, best demarcated in larger arteries because of their thicker muscular layer and less well in veins. The intimal layer of both arteries and veins typically have a brightly echogenic appearance.

APPLICATIONS IN INTERVENTIONAL RADIOLOGY

IVUS is an important complement to conventional angiography and has several applications in vascular interventions. Assessment of veins using IVUS can provide valuable information regarding the presence of venous stenosis in real time as well as the relationship with immediately adjacent structures, important in the setting of stenosis attributable to external compression, such as in May-Thurner syndrome. Additionally, IVUS can provide important information for the characterization of intraluminal thrombus in the setting of deep venous thrombosis (DVT), and can aid in the differentiation between acute and chronic thrombus and therefore effect therapy. Furthermore, in patients with recanalized DVT, IVUS can demonstrate trabeculations, bands, webs, and spurs that may be difficult to detect using venography alone. IVUS allows for the bedside placement and retrieval of IVC filters, particularly in patients with intravenous iodinated contrast allergy, pregnancy, those patients too critically ill for transport to the angiography suite, and morbidly obese patients whose weight exceeds limits of the fluoroscopy table. IVUS has also been used to guide direct puncture from IVC to the portal vein during direct intrahepatic portocaval shunt (DIPS) creation for the treatment of intractable ascites and variceal bleeding. On the arterial side, IVUS can be used during angioplasty and stenting, as well as percutaneous balloon fenestration in type B aortic dissection.

VENOUS THROMBOEMBOLISM

Iliac vein compression (May-Thurner) syndrome is an increasingly recognized cause of acute and chronic venous thromboembolism and occurs in the setting of compression of the left iliac vein by the overlying right iliac artery. Anatomic compression of the left iliac vein and chronic, repetitive injury to the venous endothelium from arterial pulsation can result in the formation of synechiae within the vein, and can progress to obstruction and even thrombosis. These patients can present with unilateral lower extremity pain, swelling, venous insufficiency, or phlegmasia.

The preferred treatment for iliac vein obstructive lesions is stent placement rather than balloon angioplasty alone.[3] This is because the fibrotic nature of venous stenosis often results in elastic recoil after balloon angioplasty. Furthermore, a residual iliac vein obstruction after venoplasty can be due to residual thrombus, stenosis, or a combination of both (Video 1). Fortunately, stent placement both expands the vein and traps residual thrombus against the vein wall, and therefore treats both residual thrombus and stenosis.[4]

IVUS has been used for both diagnosis and treatment in the setting of iliac vein compression. Accurate measurement of the degree of stenosis is important for appropriate sizing of a venous stent to be placed after venoplasty. IVUS provides an accurate measurement of the degree of iliac vein stenosis, while venography alone can underestimate stenosis by 30% (Fig. 1).[5]

In a retrospective series of 16 patients with the presumptive diagnosis of May-Thurner syndrome based on presenting symptoms and reported by Forauer and colleagues,[6] IVUS demonstrated the cause of vessel compression in all 16 patients. More importantly, IVUS findings influenced the endovascular management of iliac vein compression in half of their patients: characterization of thrombus as acute or chronic on IVUS influenced the decision to attempt adjunct pharmacologic thrombolysis or mechanical thrombectomy; incomplete expansion and apposition on IVUS resulted in additional stent deployment or further dilation of deployed stents; visualization of the guidewire in the residual venous lumen resulted in and selection of larger-diameter angioplasty balloons.

BEDSIDE INFERIOR VENA CAVA FILTER PLACEMENT

Inferior vena cava (IVC) filters have long been used in the setting of venous thromboembolism for the prevention of fatal pulmonary embolism, commonly performed percutaneously in the

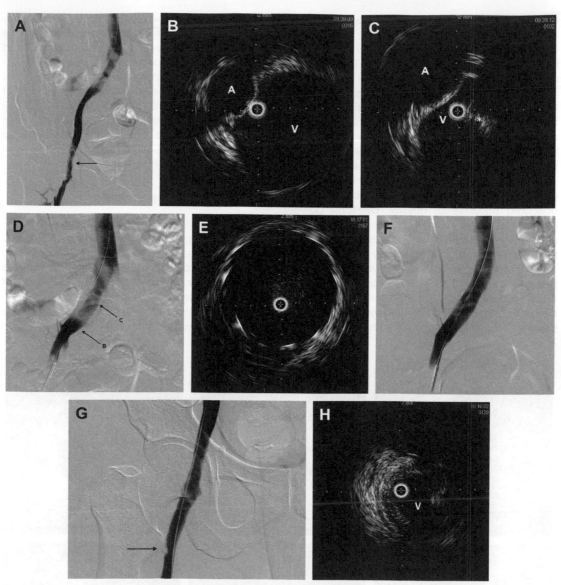

Fig. 1. A 47-year-old woman with subacute left femoral DVT. (*A*) Left iliofemoral venogram through left popliteal vein access with patient prone. Image after overnight catheter-directed thrombolysis shows residual acute on chronic DVT in the left common femoral vein (*arrow*) as well as decreased density of the common iliac vein (*asterisk*), representing chronic changes because of compression by the crossing right common iliac artery. Poor outflow as a result of this lesion likely contributed to the patient's development of acute femoral DVT. (*B*) IVUS shows a widely patent distal common iliac vein (V) with adjacent common iliac artery (A). (*C*) IVUS probe within the mid left common iliac vein (V) being compressed by the crossing right common iliac artery (*asterisk*). (*D*) Digital subtraction angiography iliofemoral venogram demonstrating levels of IVUS probe positioning at (*arrows*) B and C. Note slightly decreased density of the mid common iliac vein segment corresponding to marked extrinsic compression seen on IVUS. (*E*) IVUS positioned within the previously stenotic mid left common iliac vein segment after stent placement. (*F*) Final venogram demonstrating widely patent left common iliac vein after stent placement. (*G*) Left femoral venogram shows changes of acute on chronic DVT in the proximal superficial femoral vein. Arrow denotes level of the IVUS image in (*H*). (*H*) IVUS probe positioned in the left superficial femoral vein (V) shows corresponding wall thickening and irregularity with trabeculations, consistent with acute on chronic DVT.

angiography suite under fluoroscopy. Vena caval filter placement can also be performed at the bedside under transabdominal duplex ultrasonography and was first described in 1998. The benefits of bedside vena caval filter placement using duplex ultrasonography include reducing the need for fluoroscopy, lowering costs, and obviating the need to transport critically ill patients to the fluoroscopy suite.[7] The procedure requires adequate visualization of the IVC at the level of the renal veins using transabdominal ultrasound, because the inferior-most renal vein/IVC junction must be visualized in real time as the undeployed filter is retracted, because its disappearance from view corresponds to the appropriate position for infrarenal filter deployment. Furthermore, the IVC diameter is measured just below the level of the inferior-most renal vein for planned infrarenal placement and can affect choice of filter device.

Transabdominal duplex ultrasound is difficult in patients in whom clear visualization of the IVC is obscured because of obesity, overlying bowel gas, or open abdominal wounds. IVUS offers an alternative method for bedside filter placement in such patients and was initially described in 1999.[8] The method for bedside vena caval filter placement using IVUS involves placement of the IVUS probe in the IVC at the level of the inferior cavoatrial junction and subsequent delineation of venous anatomic landmarks using a pullback

technique. The feasibility of filter placement by IVUS alone depends on the identification of the right atrium, hepatic veins, renal veins, and common iliac vein confluence because identification of the correct location for filter deployment depends on accurate localization of the origin of the inferior-most renal vein (**Fig. 2**). IVUS-directed placement of IVC filters has been shown to be a safe, feasible, and accurate alternative to conventional fluoroscopic and transabdominal ultrasound–directed methods.[9]

AORTIC DISSECTION FENESTRATION

Aortic dissection frequently results in life-threatening organ ischemia, which is associated with high mortality. Fenestration of the dissection membrane is one therapeutic option in patients with type B dissection with mesenteric, renal, or peripheral ischemia or patients with type A dissection with persistent mesenteric, renal, or peripheral ischemia after surgical repair (Video 2). Delineation

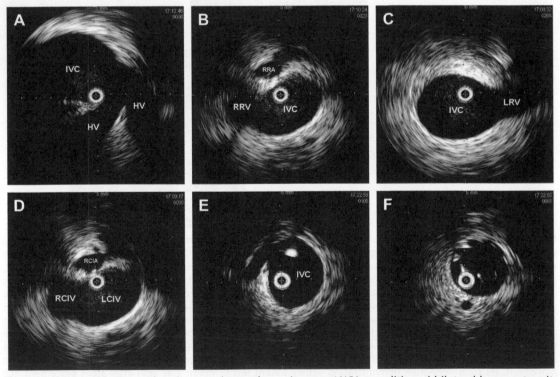

Fig. 2. A 61-year-old man with pulmonary hemorrhage due to c-ANCA vasculitis and bilateral lower extremity DVT, for IVC filter placement. Renal insufficiency precluded use of iodinated contrast. The feasibility of filter placement by IVUS alone depends on the identification of the right atrium, hepatic vein confluence, origins of the right and left renal veins, and common iliac vein confluence. Identification of the correct location for filter deployment depends on accurate localization of the origin of the inferior-most renal vein. (*A*) Hepatic vein (HV) confluence. (*B*) Origin of the right renal vein (RRV). Note right renal artery (RRA) crossing anteriorly. (*C*) Origin of the left renal vein (LRV). (*D*) Common iliac vein (CIV) confluence. (*E*) Post filter deployment images demonstrate the echogenic filter apex positioned in the IVC at the level of the RRV origin. (*F*) Echogenic metallic legs of deployed filter.

of the extension of the dissection flap and the relationship of the true and false lumen to side branches is important for understanding the altered hemodynamics in these patients and ultimately determining optimal treatment (Video 3).

IVUS is useful for guidance of percutaneous fenestration of a dissection flap. It is typically performed by transfemoral approach and involves puncture of the intimal flap with a needle-catheter combination and subsequent passage of a guidewire across the flap. A balloon catheter is then advanced over the guidewire. Particularly in patients with significant renal dysfunction, the use of IVUS can reduce the amount of iodinated contrast material used.[10]

DIPS

IVUS has been used in the guidance of direct IVC-to–portal vein puncture for creation of DIPS for the treatment of intractable ascites and variceal bleeding. A transfemorally placed transducer is positioned in the IVC and used for real-time guidance of the IVC-to–portal vein puncture of an access needle that has been passed from a transjugular approach. Primary patency of the shunt has been shown to be greater than that with conventional transjugular intrahepatic portosystemic shunt.[11]

LIMITATIONS

As with conventional ultrasound, IVUS suffers from several image artifacts that are important to recognize and understand to allow for more effective use. The guide wire over which the IVUS probe is advanced causes image dropout of approximately 15° in the location of the wire. Careful flushing with saline is required to avoid shadowing or distortion from air bubbles. The development of dual-channel catheters allow for removal of the wire, which alleviates this problem. Acoustic shadowing can occur from several causes, including calcification, stent struts, and IVC filters. Reverberation artifact can affect IVUS images, as it can with conventional ultrasound, resulting in concentric circular echoes equidistant from the probe.[2]

SUMMARY

Advances in IVUS technology may further broaden the capabilities and applications of this already useful tool. For example, color imaging and 3-dimensional imaging may further improve the ability to accurately characterize intraluminal thrombus and luminal borders. Color imaging detects differences between sequential axial images to construct a color map depicting areas of flow, which may prove useful for distinguishing between partial and complete thrombosis.[12] Three-dimensional reconstructions over a vessel segment can be used to create a longitudinal image of the vessel. Through such advancements, the benefits of IVUS guidance in endovascular interventions may further increase their utility in interventional radiology.

VIDEOS

Videos related to this article can be found online at http://dx.doi.org/10.1016/j.cult.2012.12.007.

REFERENCES

1. Lee JT, White RA. Basics of intravascular ultrasound: an essential tool for the endovascular surgeon. Semin Vasc Surg 2004;17(2):110–8.
2. McLafferty RB. The role of intravascular ultrasound in venous thromboembolism. Semin Intervent Radiol 2012;29:10–5.
3. Semba CP, Dake MD. Catheter directed thrombolysis for iliofemoral venous thrombosis. Semin Vasc Surg 1996;9:26–33.
4. Vedantham S, Thorpe PE, Cardella JF, et al. Quality improvement guidelines for the treatment of lower extremity deep vein thrombosis with use of endovascular thrombus removal. J Vasc Interv Radiol 2006; 17:435–48.
5. Neglen P, Raju S. Intravascular ultrasound scan evaluation of the obstructed vein. J Vasc Surg 2002;35(4):694–700.
6. Forauer AR, Gemmete JJ, Dasika NL, et al. Intravascular ultrasound in the diagnosis and treatment of iliac vein compression (May-Thurner) syndrome. J Vasc Interv Radiol 2002;13:523–7.
7. Neuzil DF, Garrard CL, Berkman RA, et al. Duplex-directed vena caval filter placement: report of initial experience. Surgery 1998;123:470–4.
8. Oppat FO, Chiou AC, Matsumura JS. Intravascular ultrasound-guided vena cava filter placement. J Endovasc Surg 1999;6(3):285–7.
9. Passman MA, Dattilo JB, Guzman RJ, et al. Bedside placement of inferior vena cava filters by using transabdominal duplex ultrasonography and intravascular ultrasound imaging. J Vasc Surg 2005;42: 1027–32.
10. Vedantham S, Picus D, Sanchez L, et al. Percutaneous management of ischemic complications in patients with type-B aortic dissection. J Vasc Interv Radiol 2003;14:181–93.
11. Petersen B, Binkert C. Intravascular ultrasound-guided direct intrahepatic portacaval shunt: midterm follow-up. J Vasc Interv Radiol 2004;15:927–38.
12. Manninen HI, Räsänen H. Intravascular ultrasound in interventional radiology. Eur Radiol 2000;10: 1754–62.

The Use of Ultrasound in Musculoskeletal Interventions

Valeriy Kheyfits, MD[a],*, Meena K. Moorthy, MD, MBA[a],
Jack Jennings, MD[b], Travis J. Hillen, MD[b]

KEYWORDS

- Musculoskeletal intervention • Joint aspiration • Iliopsoas bursa • Iliopsoas tendinopathy
- Neuroma • Plantar fascia • Greater trochanteric bursa • Soft tissue mass biopsy

KEY POINTS

- Ultrasound is a readily available, cost-effective method to diagnose and treat many disorders of the musculoskeletal system.
- Uses include, but are not limited to, injection of medication, aspiration of bursae or cysts, biopsy, and treatment of calcific tendinosis.
- It is a safe modality for children and during pregnancy.

 A video of ultrasound-guided barbotage of calcific tendinosis of the rotator cuff accompanies this article.

INTRODUCTION

Ultrasound (US) is a widely available, inexpensive modality for performing a variety of musculoskeletal-themed imaging-guided interventions that address common problems and concerns frequently encountered by patients seen in the orthopedic, physical medicine/rehabilitation, and podiatrist clinics. One of the major advantages of US is that it can be used for both diagnostic and interventional purposes. A diagnosis can be confirmed or obtained, and treatment can be provided, often on the same visit, with a minimum of inconvenience to both the patient and the referring clinician.

In addition to being a safe modality for pregnant women and children/adolescents, sonography has the added benefit in imaging of postsurgical patients, in whom magnetic resonance (MR) imaging or computed tomography may falter because of the presence of hardware. The ability to perform dynamic imaging is another benefit of sonography, and it can be used during procedures to optimize the approach and minimize the risk of complications.

US TECHNIQUE

To successfully perform US-guided procedures, the clinician must be familiar with the basics of US imaging, able to optimize sonographic technique to visualize the abnormality or joint space, and be thoroughly versed in the appropriate musculoskeletal anatomy, including surface anatomy. In general, linear probes with the highest frequency (7–12 MHz) to produce adequate penetration are preferred. For lesions situated deeper or in larger patients, a curvilinear low-frequency probe may need to be used.

US scale should be optimized for best visualization at the needed depth. Doppler US is useful for mapping out adjacent vessels to avoid vascular injury during the procedure or to determine the vascularity of a lesion before biopsy. It is important

[a] Department of Imaging Sciences, University of Rochester Medical Center, 601 Elmwood Avenue, Rochester, NY 14642, USA; [b] Musculoskeletal Section, Mallinckrodt Institute of Radiology, Washington University School of Medicine in St. Louis, 510 South Kingshighway Boulevard, St Louis, MO 63110, USA
* Corresponding author.
E-mail address: valeriy_kheyfits@urmc.rochester.edu

Ultrasound Clin 8 (2013) 191–200
http://dx.doi.org/10.1016/j.cult.2012.12.013
1556-858X/13/$ – see front matter © 2013 Elsevier Inc. All rights reserved.

to avoid introduction of air into the tissues during the procedure, because air bubbles reduce visibility and may completely obscure the target.

Choices of steroid medications usually include methylprednisolone, triamcinolone, or betamethasone. Betamethasone is preferred for the more superficial injections, because it is less likely to produce skin discoloration. Dosage varies with physician preference and patient's condition, but, in general, 40 to 80 mg of triamcinolone or methylprednisolone or 6 to 12 mg of betamethasone are used.

Long acting local anesthetic such as bupivacaine (0.25% or 0.5%) may be administered in conjunction with the steroid.

INTERVENTIONS

US-guided musculoskeletal interventions include but are not limited to:

- Injection of medication to treat arthritis, tendinosis, neuromas, and overuse syndromes
- Identification and removal of foreign bodies
- Needle aspiration of calcific tendonitis
- Needle aspiration of bursae, ganglions, and cysts
- Diagnostic and/or therapeutic needle aspiration for crystalline arthropathy or septic arthritis
- Platelet-rich plasma (PRP) and autologous blood injection
- Soft tissue mass biopsy

PRP

PRP is derived from centrifuging whole blood, resulting in a highly cellular component of plasma containing numerous growth factors. Injecting PRP directly into the site of injury is a practice that is gaining popularity in the treatment of ligament and tendon tears.[1]

Soft Tissue Mass Biopsy

A request to biopsy a soft tissue mass of musculoskeletal origin using US is a common occurrence in clinical practice. The differential diagnosis varies from benign causes such as lipoma to malignant causes including metastases and soft tissue sarcoma. Before biopsy of the soft tissue mass, if it is most likely a sarcoma, the appropriate approach to biopsy should be discussed with the oncologic surgeon in case limb-sparing surgery is a surgical option.

Local anesthesia is achieved with 1% lidocaine before biopsy. US is used to evaluate the mass for viable tumor because many large masses have areas of central necrosis. Once a viable area of tumor has been localized, a spring-loaded core biopsy needle is used to obtain multiple samples that are delivered to pathology (**Fig. 1**).

UPPER EXTREMITY
Shoulder

US interventions in the shoulder are many, because the joint is commonly affected by injury, rotator cuff disorders, and arthropathies.

Subacromial/subdeltoid bursal injection
The subacromial-subdeltoid (SASD) bursa can be inflamed in conditions such as rheumatoid arthritis, gout, calcium pyrophosphate dihydrate deposition disease (CPPD), or pyogenic infection. More commonly, it is inflamed secondary to shoulder impingement syndrome.

When injecting the SASD bursa it is essential to first rule out septic bursitis and a rotator cuff tear, because local injection of corticosteroids is contraindicated in these conditions.

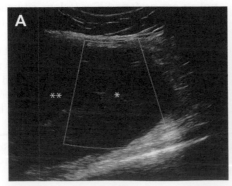 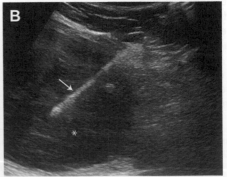

Fig. 1. A 52-year-old woman with painful posterior thigh mass most consistent with sarcoma. (*A*) A large posterior thigh mass containing both solid (*asterisk*) and necrotic areas (*double asterisk*). (*B*) The biopsy needle (*arrow*) within the solid (*asterisk*) component of the mass. This lesion at pathology is a myxofibrosarcoma.

Injection of the SASD bursa is performed with patients seated, and their arm positioned behind their back with the elbows bent. Imaging through the coracoacromial window provides visualization of the bursa and adjacent structures. The needle is inserted horizontally, and aspiration of effusion is performed. In our institution, we typically use a 22-G spinal needle to both aspirate and inject the bursa with a steroid-lidocaine suspension.[2]

Calcific tendinopathy barbotage
Calcium hydroxyapatite deposition in the substance of a tendon is a common cause of shoulder pain, primarily affecting young to middle-aged individuals, with a slight female predilection. In the shoulder, the supraspinatus tendon is most commonly affected, followed by the infraspinatus and subscapularis tendons.

Percutaneous fragmentation and aspiration of calcium deposits can often relieve symptoms in patients with pain refractory to nonsteroidal antiinflammatory drugs (NSAIDs).

The patient is usually in a seated position, and a horizontal approach along the anteroposterior axis is favored for the needle path. US is used to identify the target calcium deposit and, under real-time US monitoring, an 18G to 22G needle is used to puncture the calcium deposit (**Fig. 2**).

A 10-mL syringe filled with a saline-lidocaine solution is used to fragment the calcium deposit, using a gentle pulse-aspiration technique. As the calcium fragments, it is partially aspirated into the syringe, where it appears as fine, grainlike particles. Some of particles are dispersed in the surrounding soft tissues and are resorbed by the body.[3,4]

Following this procedure, a small amount of steroid/anesthetic mixture is injected into the resulting cavity and into the SASD bursa to decrease inflammation and pain.

Joint injection
Injection of an antiinflammatory medication, such as a corticosteroid, into a joint is typically done to reduce pain and inflammation from conditions such as arthritis and tendinosis.

Caution must be used when injecting a corticosteroid, because this class of medication can cause skin and/or fat necrosis and atrophy, degeneration of the tendon, and breakdown of cartilage.

Glenohumeral joint Injection of the glenohumeral joint is a commonly performed procedure. The patient is usually placed in a posterior oblique position, with the affected shoulder projecting upwards. The transducer is placed transversely to visualize the glenohumeral joint at the level of the coracoid process. The needle is then placed from a lateral approach into the joint under the subscapularis tendon. Lidocaine (1%) is used to achieve local anesthesia. In our institution, we typically use a 22-G spinal needle to enter the joint.[5,6]

Acromioclavicular joint Injection of the acromioclavicular (AC) joint is usually performed with the patient in a sitting position. Lidocaine (1%) is used to achieve local anesthesia. In our institution, we typically use a 22-G, 34-mm needle to enter the joint.

Tendon injection
In the shoulder, inflammation of the synovium of a tendon sheath usually involves the biceps tendon. This injury is commonly a result of overuse or acute trauma.

Injection of the biceps tendon for tenosynovitis is typically performed with the patient seated, hands resting in the lap (internally rotated). The point of entry is the bicipital groove, which is located about 25 mm caudal to the anterolateral margin of the acromion.[7]

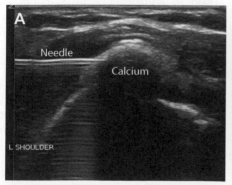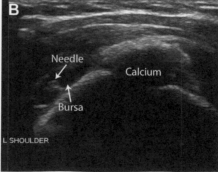

Fig. 2. A 69-year-old woman with left shoulder pain who had extensive calcific tendinitis on radiographs. US-guided supraspinatus calcific tendinitis barbotage and subacromial-subdeltoid (SASD) bursa injection were performed. (*A*) The needle entering the supraspinatus calcific tendinitis lesion (calcium) parallel to the US beam. (*B*) The injection of the SASD bursa after barbotage.

Lidocaine (1%) is used to achieve local anesthesia. Using US guidance, a 25-G needle is inserted using an anterior approach, with the needle entering the skin at 30°, and directed parallel to the bicipital groove (**Fig. 3**). A small amount of anesthetic/steroid suspension should be injected in a peritendinous distribution. Care must be taken not to inject directly into the tendon.

Cyst aspiration

AC joint synovial cyst Degenerative changes are common in the AC joint, and can lead to formation of synovial cysts. These cysts occasionally communicate with the SASD bursa in the setting of concomitant rotator cuff disorders.

Paralabral cyst Paralabral cysts are collections of joint fluid that develop secondary to tears of the labrum. They can occur in any location around the glenoid. The cyst itself is usually painless, but can become symptomatic as the cysts become large. Large cysts can impinge on the nerves supplying the shoulder musculature, leading to muscle atrophy, weakness, and pain.

Using US guidance, paralabral or AC joint synovial cyst can be aspirated to provide symptom relief. After administering local anesthetic, a larger-gauge needle (18 or 20 G) is used to puncture and aspirate the cyst. Following this procedure, a small amount of steroid is injected into the resultant cavity, to reduce inflammation and risk of reoccurrence (**Fig. 4**).[8,9]

Elbow

The elbow joint can become painful and inflamed in a variety of conditions such as osteoarthritis, rheumatoid arthritis, and crystalline arthropathies. Pain and swelling can also be a result of trauma or infection.

Joint injection/aspiration

Injection or aspiration of the elbow joint is performed with the patient supine or seated and the elbow flexed to 45°, with the hand in a neutral position. Lidocaine (1%) is used to achieve local anesthesia. A lateral approach is favored, thus avoiding the ulnar nerve. In our institution, we typically use an 18-G or 20-G needle for aspiration, and a 22-G needle for injection of corticosteroids (**Fig. 5**).[5,6]

Lateral epicondylitis

This painful condition is thought to be secondary to chronic degenerative changes at the origin of the extensor carpi radialis brevis, with tiny tears in the tendon attachment at the elbow.

Steroid injection for lateral epicondylitis is performed with the patient supine or seated and the elbow flexed at 45°, resting on the patient's side. The wrist should be pronated. Lidocaine (1%) is used to achieve local anesthesia. A 25-G needle is used, held at 90° to the lateral epicondyle and advanced under US guidance to within 1 to 2 mm of the bone.[10,11]

PRP injection for partial tendon tears

Local injection of PRP into injured tissue is a practice that is gaining popularity. It is thought that the growth factors contained in PRP can accelerate the healing process by promoting collagen scar formation.

The elbow is a common site of tendon and ligament injuries, largely caused by repetitive microtrauma, especially in athletes.

Local anesthesia can be achieved with 1% lidocaine, or bupivacaine with epinephrine. The injured tendon is identified with US, and a 22-G needle is used to administer 2 to 3 mL of PRP using a peppering technique that involves a single cutaneous portal, but multiple fenestrations/injections of the tendon.[2]

Olecranon bursa aspiration

Olecranon bursitis is commonly caused by repetitive trauma, although it can also be seen with rheumatoid arthritis and crystalline arthropathies. The fluid-filled bursa is readily identified on physical examination, because it is a superficial structure. The bursa can be secondarily infected, in which case aspiration can be performed, but injection with corticosteroids is contraindicated.

Aspiration of the olecranon bursa is performed with the patient supine and the elbow flexed as much as the patient can tolerate. An 18-G needle

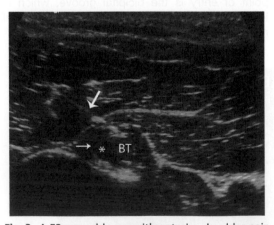

Fig. 3. A 52-year-old man with anterior shoulder pain most consistent with biceps tenosynovitis. US image showing needle placement (*large arrow*) within the extra-articular biceps tendon sheath (*small arrow*) just superficial to the biceps tendon (BT) with filling of the biceps tendon sheath (*asterisk*).

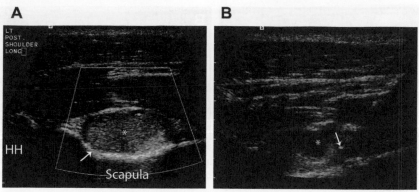

Fig. 4. A 30-year-old right-hand-dominant professional baseball pitcher with left shoulder pain who had an MR examination showing a paralabral cyst. (*A*) A large spinoglenoid notch (*arrow*) paralabral cyst (*asterisk*) containing echogenic debris. The humeral head (HH) and scapula are also labeled. (*B*) The needle (*arrow*) within a partially aspirated, complex-appearing paralabral cyst (*asterisk*).

is used to enter and aspirate the fluid-filled bursa (**Fig. 6**).[11,12]

Wrist

The wrist is commonly involved with such processes as arthropathy, carpal tunnel syndrome, tenosynovitis, and ganglion cysts.

Aspiration/injection of ganglion cyst

The most common soft tissue mass in the distal upper extremity, a ganglion cyst is a collection of sticky, mucoid fluid that occurs adjacent or attached to the joint capsule or tendon sheath. These masses can occur in any joint, but are often seen in the scapholunate interval, dorsum of the wrist, and in the fingers. Ganglion cysts can become large and painful, and thus treatment is often required.

The patient is usually supine or sitting, with the wrist and hand resting at the side, and with the target surface facing upward. Lidocaine (1%) is used to achieve local anesthesia. Using US guidance, an 18-G to 22-G needle is inserted into the cyst, which is then aspirated. Following this procedure, a small amount of steroid can be injected into the cavity to reduce inflammation.[13,14]

Injection for tenosynovitis

Tenosynovitis is inflammation of the synovium surrounding the tendon sheath, and can cause pain, swelling, and decreased range of motion. Tenosynovitis can result from injury, infection, arthropathy, or repetitive microtrauma.

The patient should be supine, with the wrist and hand resting at the side, with the target surface facing upward. Lidocaine (1%) is used to achieve local anesthesia. Using US guidance, a 25-G needle is inserted parallel to the affected tendon, and a small amount of steroid/anesthetic suspension is injected into the tendon sheath. Care must be taken not to inject directly into the tendon.[13,14]

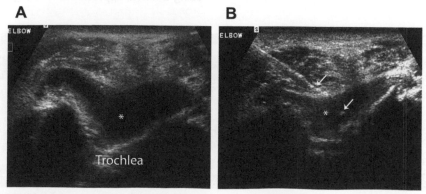

Fig. 5. A 60-year-old woman with left elbow pain and swelling. (*A*) A medium elbow effusion (*asterisk*) superficial to the humeral trochlea. (*B*) The needle (*arrow*) within a partially decompressed effusion (*asterisk*). Analysis of the fluid showed crystals consistent with a gout flair.

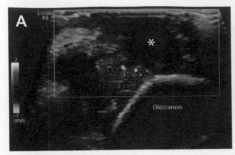
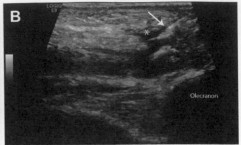

Fig. 6. A 74-year-old man with elbow swelling and cellulitis. (*A*) Fluid (*asterisk*) within the inflamed olecranon bursa. (*B*) A needle (*arrow*) within the decompressed olecranon bursa (*asterisk*). The aspirate grew abundant *Staphylococcus aureus*.

LOWER EXTREMITY

Hip

The hip joint is commonly involved with such conditions as trauma, arthritis, and injury from repetitive microtrauma.

Joint injection/aspiration

Hip joint effusion is common, and can cause pain and decreased range of motion. In many cases, the fluid is infected, and aspiration can be performed for both diagnostic and therapeutic purposes. The hip joint fluid usually accumulates in the anterior recess, and is readily identifiable by US.

Aspiration of the hip joint effusion is performed with the patient in the supine position and the transducer positioned along the axis of the femoral neck to evaluate the anterior recess. Lidocaine (1%) is used to achieve local anesthesia. A 16-G to 18-G needle is used, and an anterolateral approach is favored, with US guidance in the longitudinal plane. The needle should be placed in the largest pocket of fluid within the anterior recess, and aspirated (**Fig. 7**). Corticosteroid injection is contraindicated if septic effusion is suspected/known.[15,16]

Iliopsoas tendon injection

Iliopsoas tendinosis can be seen with inflammatory arthropathy, overuse injury, trauma, or in the setting of total hip arthroplasty.

Snapping hip syndrome is characterized by a snapping sensation when the hip is extended and flexed. In the extra-articular type, the iliotibial band, tensor fascia lata, or gluteus medius tendon is thickened, and catches on the greater trochanter with motion. In the intra-articular type, which is most common, the iliopsoas tendon catches in the anterior inferior iliac spine.

Injection of the iliopsoas tendon is performed with the patient in the supine position, using a lateral approach at the level of the iliopectineal eminence. Lidocaine (1%) is used to achieve local anesthesia. A 22-G needle is used to inject steroid/anesthetic suspension into the iliopsoas bursa and/or in a peritendinous distribution. Care must be taken not to inject directly into the tendon.[17,18]

Aspiration/injection of the iliopsoas bursa

Aspiration or injection of the iliopsoas bursa is performed with the patient in the supine position, using a lateral approach with US guidance in the

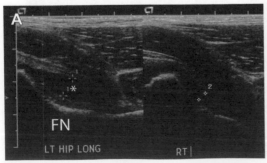
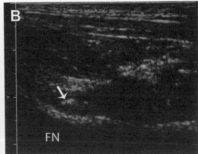

Fig. 7. A 5-year-old boy with acute-onset left hip pain. (*A*) A large left hip effusion (*asterisk*) with no right hip effusion. (*B*) A decompressed left joint following needle (*arrow*) aspiration. Hematologic and hip fluid laboratory findings were consistent with toxic synovitis. FN, femoral neck.

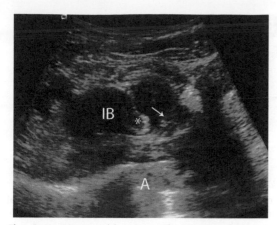

Fig. 8. A 55-year-old man with anterior hip pain following total hip arthroplasty. The US image shows the needle (*arrow*) within a distended iliopsoas bursa (IB) surrounding the iliopsoas tendon (*asterisk*) superficial to the acetabulum (A).

axial plane. Lidocaine (1%) is used to achieve local anesthesia. A 16-G to 18-G needle is used for aspiration of the bursa, whereas a 22-G needle is usually used for injections (**Fig. 8**).[15,16]

Aspiration/injection of the greater trochanteric bursa

Trochanteric bursitis presents with pain along the lateral aspect of the hip with activity. It can occur secondary to overuse injury, snapping hip syndrome, or rheumatoid arthritis.

Aspiration or injection of the greater trochanteric bursa is performed with the patient in the lateral decubitus position, with the affected hip facing upward. A lateral approach is used with US guidance in the axial or sagittal plane. Lidocaine (1%) is used to achieve local anesthesia. A 16-G to 18-G needle is used for aspiration of the bursa, whereas a 22-G needle may be used for injection (**Fig. 9**).[15,16]

Knee

The knee is a common site of involvement in acute trauma, overuse injury, and arthropathy.

Joint injection/aspiration

Intra-articular aspiration or injection of the knee is performed with the patient in a supine position, with the knee either fully extended or slightly flexed and supported by a pillow in the popliteal space. Lidocaine (1%) is used to achieve local anesthesia. An 18-G to 20-G needle is used for aspirations and a 25-G needle may be used for injections. The approach can be lateral, medial, or anterior.[19]

Parameniscal cyst aspiration

Parameniscal cysts can form as a complication of meniscal tears, and can present with pain and limited range of motion. These cysts can form adjacent to the lateral or medial meniscus, and generally have a direct communication with the meniscal tear.

Aspiration of a parameniscal cyst is performed with the patient in a supine position, with the knee either fully extended or slightly flexed and supported by a pillow in the popliteal space. Lidocaine (1%) is used to achieve local anesthesia. A 16-G needle is used to access the cyst under US guidance and aspirate to dryness. The approach can be medial or lateral depending on the location of the cyst, and the needle should enter the cyst at an oblique angle (45° ± 15°) to achieve maximum aspiration (**Fig. 10**).[20]

Baker cyst aspiration

Aspiration of a Baker cyst is performed with the patient prone, and the knee extended. Lidocaine (1%) is used to achieve local anesthesia. Using US guidance, a 16-G needle is used to access the cyst and aspirate to dryness (**Fig. 11**).[21]

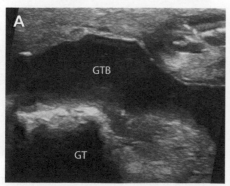
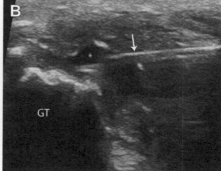

Fig. 9. A 54-year-old woman with lateral thigh pain following hip replacement. (A) A very distended greater trochanteric bursa (GTB) superficial to the greater trochanter (GT). (B) Decompression of the GTB (*asterisk*) following needle (*arrow*) aspiration.

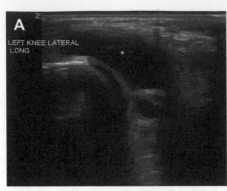
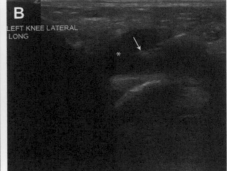

Fig. 10. A 49-year-old woman with lateral knee pain found to have a lateral meniscus tear with a parameniscal cyst. (*A*) A large lateral parameniscal cyst (*asterisk*). (*B*) The needle (*arrow*) within the parameniscal cyst (*asterisk*).

Ankle

Joint injection/aspiration

An ankle joint effusion can occur in the setting of trauma, arthropathy, connective tissue disease, or synovitis. Patients may present with pain and/or limited range of motion.

Aspiration or injection of the ankle joint is performed with the patient supine and the ankle in neutral position. Lidocaine (1%) is used to achieve local anesthesia. Under US guidance, a 25-G needle is inserted into the tibiotalar articulation, typically using an anteromedial approach.[22]

Tenosynovitis injection

In the ankle, inflammation of the synovium of a tendon sheath usually involves the Achilles or peroneal tendons, although the Achilles tendon possesses a paratenon rather than a true tendon sheath. This injury is commonly a result of overuse or acute trauma.

Injection of the Achilles paratenon for tenosynovitis is performed with the patient prone, with the affected foot extended over the edge of the examination table. Lidocaine (1%) is used to achieve local anesthesia. Using US guidance, a 25-G needle in a lateral approach is used to inject a small amount of anesthetic/steroid suspension in a peritendinous distribution. Care must be taken not to inject directly into the tendon. For tibialis posterior or peroneal tendon sheath injections, medial and lateral approaches are used, respectively (**Fig. 12**).[23]

Ganglion cyst aspiration

As in the upper extremity, a ganglion cyst may cause symptoms from mass effect on adjacent structures, including pain and weakness, particularly if involving the tarsal tunnel.

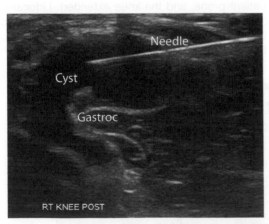

Fig. 11. A 51-year-old woman with painful, palpable swelling in the popliteal fossa. US image from a popliteal/Baker cyst aspiration showing the needle entering a comma-shaped fluid collection between the medial head of the gastrocnemius (gastroc) and the semimembranosus.

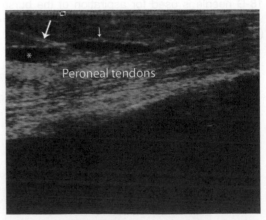

Fig. 12. Injection of the peroneal tendon sheath in a young woman with lateral ankle pain. The needle (*large arrow*) is superficial to the peroneal tendons but deep to the peroneal retinaculum (*small arrow*) with filling of the tendon sheath (*asterisk*).

Aspiration of a ganglion cyst in the ankle is performed with the patient prone or supine, depending on the location of the mass. The target area should be facing upward. Lidocaine (1%) is used to achieve local anesthesia. Using US guidance, an 18-G to 22-G needle is inserted into the cyst, which is then aspirated. Following this procedure, a small amount of steroid/anesthetic suspension can be injected into the cavity to reduce inflammation (**Fig. 13**).[24]

Foot

Subtalar joint injection

The subtalar joint can be involved in a variety of conditions such as arthropathy, synovitis, coalition, or trauma. Symptoms such as pain and decreased range of motion can significantly affect a patient's mobility.

Intra-articular injection of the subtalar joint is performed with the patient prone and the ankle in neutral position. Using a posterolateral approach, a 25-G needle is inserted under US monitoring toward the center of the talus.[24,25]

Neuroma injection

A plantar neuroma (also known as Morton neuroma) is a benign condition in which there is fibrous tissue/scar formation around an intermetatarsal plantar nerve. Morton neuromas occur secondary to repetitive stress/microtrauma, and are most common in the third or fourth intermetatarsal space. Mass effect from the neuroma can lead to pain and numbness.

Injection is performed with the patient supine and the knee flexed and supported with a pillow in the popliteal space. The ankle and foot should be in a neutral position. The neuroma should be identified under US monitoring, and 1% lidocaine is used to achieve local anesthesia. A 25-G needle is inserted into the web space or dorsum of the foot at a 45° angle to the neuroma. A slow injection of steroid/anesthetic suspension (preferably betamethasone) is done, taking care not to inject the fat pad at the base of the foot.[24]

Intermetatarsal bursa injection/aspiration

Injection or aspiration of an intermetatarsal bursa is performed with the patient supine and the knee flexed and supported with a pillow in the popliteal space. The ankle and foot should be in a neutral position. Lidocaine (1%) is used to achieve local anesthesia. A 20-G needle is inserted into the web space or dorsum of the foot, with placement in the bursa confirmed with US monitoring. Once the bursa has been aspirated to dryness, a small amount of steroid/anesthetic suspension can be injected into the cavity to reduce inflammation.[24]

Plantar fascia injection

Plantar fasciitis is generally a result of overuse, and can be painful. When the pain is not relieved by rest and NSAIDs, local injection of corticosteroids may be considered.

Injection is performed with the patient in a lateral recumbent position, with the affected foot down. The point of maximum tenderness along the medial aspect of the foot can be determined with gentle pressure on the US probe. A 22-G needle is then inserted at 90° from a medial approach or from a posterior approach slightly superficial to the plantar fascia. A slow injection of steroid/anesthetic suspension should be performed as the needle is withdrawn, taking care to avoid injecting into the fat pad at the base of the foot.[26]

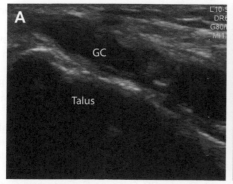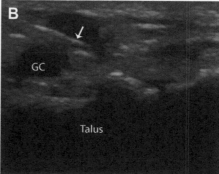

Fig. 13. A 42-year-old woman with an anterolateral foot mass and pain most consistent with ganglion cyst. US images show the preprocedural appearance of a multilobulated ganglion cyst (GC) arising from the dorsolateral talonavicular joint (*A*) and the intraprocedural appearance of the cyst, which is decreased in size with the needle (*arrow*) in place (*B*). Reduction in the patient's pain was achieved after 1.5 mL of thick serous fluid was obtained from the cyst.

Plantar fibroma injection

A plantar fibroma is a benign nodule composed of collagen tissue, arising in the plantar fascia. Depending on its location, a plantar fibroma can cause pain when walking or standing.

Steroid injection into a plantar fibroma is usually performed with the patient in a lateral recumbent position, with the affected foot down. A 22-G needle is then inserted at 90° from a medial approach or from a posterior approach slightly superficial to the plantar fascia. A slow injection of steroid/anesthetic suspension should be performed as the needle is withdrawn, taking care to avoid injecting into the fat pad at the base of the foot.[24,26]

VIDEO

Video related to this article can be found online at http://dx.doi.org/10.1016/j.cult.2012.12.013.

REFERENCES

1. Sanchez M, Guadilla J, Andia I. Ultrasound-guided platelet-rich plasma injections for the treatment of osteoarthritis of the hip. Available at: www.rheumatology.oxfordjournals.org. (Accessed June 11, 2012).

2. Chen M, Lew HL, Hsu TC, et al. Ultrasound-guided shoulder injections in the treatment of subacromial bursitis. Am J Phys Med Rehabil 2006;85(1):31–5.

3. Rima A, Cardinal E, Bureau NJ, et al. Calcific shoulder tendinitis: treatment with modified US-guided fine-needle technique. Radiology 2001;221:455–61.

4. Farin PU, Rasanen H, Jaroma H, et al. Rotator cuff calcifications: treatment with ultrasound-guided percutaneous needle aspiration and lavage. Skeletal Radiol 1996;25:551–4.

5. Lin H, Learch T, White E, et al. Emergency joint aspiration: a guide for radiologists on call. Radiographics 2009;29:1139–58.

6. Fessell DP, Jacobson JA, Craig J, et al. Using sonography to reveal and aspirate joint effusions. AJR Am J Roentgenol 2000;174:1353–62.

7. Smith J, Finnoff J. Diagnostic and interventional musculoskeletal ultrasound: part 2 clinical applications. PM R 2009;1:162–77.

8. Hiller A, Miller JD, Zeller JL. Acromioclavicular joint cyst formation. Clin Anat 2010;23:145–52.

9. Bathia N, Malanga G. Ultrasound-guided aspiration and corticosteroid injection in the management of a paralabral ganglion cyst. PM R 2009;1:1041–4.

10. McShane J, Shah VN, Nazarian LN. Sonographically guided percutaneous needle tenotomy for treatment of common extensor tendinosis in the elbow. Is a corticosteroid necessary? J Ultrasound Med 2008;27:1137–44.

11. Cardone D, Tallia A. Diagnostic and therapeutic injection of the elbow region. Am Fam Physician 2002;66(11):2097–100.

12. Louis LJ. Musculoskeletal ultrasound intervention: principles and advances. Radiol Clin North Am 2008;46:515–33.

13. Tallia A, Cardone D. Diagnostic and therapeutic injection of the wrist and hand region. Am Fam Physician 2003;67(4):745–50.

14. Wysocki R, Biswas D, Bayne C. Injection therapy in the management of musculoskeletal injuries: hand and wrist. Oper Tech Sports Med 2012;20:132–41 © Elsevier Inc.

15. Rowbotham E, Grainger A. Ultrasound-guided intervention around the hip joint. AJR Am J Roentgenol 2011;197:W122–7.

16. Cardone D, Tallia A. Diagnostic and therapeutic injection of the hip and knee. Am Fam Physician 2003;67(10):2147–52.

17. Blankenbaker D, De Smet A, Keene J. Sonography of the iliopsoas tendon and injection of the iliopsoas bursa for diagnosis and management of the painful snapping hip. Skeletal Radiol 2006;35:565–71.

18. Adler R, Buly R, Ambrose R. Diagnostic and therapeutic use of sonography-guided iliopsoas peritendinous injections. AJR Am J Roentgenol 2005;185:940–3.

19. Park Y, Sang CL, Hee-Seung N. Comparison of sonographically guided intra-articular injections at 3 different sites of the knee. J Ultrasound Med 2011;30:1669–76.

20. MacMahon PJ, Brennan DD, Duke D. Ultrasound-guided percutaneous drainage of meniscal cysts: preliminary clinical experience. Clin Radiol 2007;62:683–7.

21. Di Santi L, Paoloni M, Ioppolo F, et al. Ultrasound-guided aspiration and corticosteroid injection of Baker's cysts in knee osteoarthritis. Am J Phys Med Rehabil 2010;89(12):970–5.

22. Roy S, Dewitz A, Paul I, et al. Ultrasound-assisted ankle arthrocentesis. Am J Emerg Med 1999;17:300–1.

23. Mehdizade A, Adler R. Sonographically guided flexor hallucis longus tendon sheath injection. J Ultrasound Med 2007;26:233–7.

24. Tallia A, Cardone D. Diagnostic and therapeutic injection of the ankle and foot. Am Fam Physician 2003;68(7):1356–62.

25. Wisniewsli S, Smith J, Patterson DG, et al. Ultrasound-guided versus nonguided tibiotalar joint and sinus tarsi injections: a cadaveric study. PM R 2010;2:277–81.

26. Brophy DP, Cunnane G, Fitzgereald O, et al. Technical report: Ultrasound guidance for injection of soft tissue lesions around the heel in chronic inflammatory arthritis. Clin Radiol 1995;50:120–2.

Ultrasonography and GPS Technology

John McGrath, MD[a], David N. Siegel, MD, FSIR[b],
David L. Waldman, MD, PhD, FACR, FSIR[c],*

KEYWORDS

- Electromagnetic navigation • Image-guided therapy • Coregistration • Ultrasonography
- Global positioning system

KEY POINTS

- Ultrasonography allows real-time guidance of percutaneous ablation and biopsy.
- Coregistration and fusion allow data from 2 separate imaging studies to be superimposed or viewed in parallel for procedural guidance.
- Electromagnetic navigation, akin to global positioning systems (GPS), allows accurate intraprocedural tracking in real time of interventional radiology tools and equipment in any imaging plane.
- Ultrasound GPS provides an improved means of incorporating the spatial resolution and information regarding lesion contrast enhancement from computed tomography or magnetic resonance, or metabolic activity on positron emission tomography imaging into the interventional radiology suite.

 Videos of needle guidance for biopsy of a right hepatic lobe lesion, of pre-procedure fusion scanning, and of targeting of a right hepatic lobe lesion using historic contrast enhanced CT accompany this article.

INTRODUCTION

The advent of image-guided, minimally invasive procedures has changed medical intervention in recent years. Many procedures in interventional radiology, including percutaneous biopsy and ablation, require accurate placement of a needle, catheter, biopsy gun, or probe.[1] Accurate placement of such tools has traditionally been limited by several factors, including the image modality chosen for guidance. Individual imaging modalities confer specific benefits and drawbacks, and the optimal operating suite would incorporate favorable elements of each. For instance, while computed tomography (CT) offers excellent inherent spatial resolution, this comes at the expense of a significant dose of radiation to the patient. Similarly,

CT and magnetic resonance (MR) offer the ability to visualize some lesions made conspicuous only following contrast administration, but such differential enhancement is usually a transient phenomenon of limited benefit during lengthy interventional radiology procedures (**Fig. 1**). Ultrasonography, however, provides real-time imaging, and does so without the use of ionizing radiation. Many lesions are unfortunately not visible on a sonogram (**Fig. 2**). Sonographic visualization of needles or trocars during biopsy or ablation is limited to a single ultrasound plane, and may be affected by needle angle. Needle tips and ablation probes may be of variable echogenicity, a potential additional limitation.[2]

Operator inability to imagine the complex 3-dimensional spatial relationship necessary for

[a] Department of Radiology, University of Rochester Medical Center, 601 Elmwood Avenue, Box 648, Rochester, NY 14642, USA; [b] Division of Vascular/Interventional Radiology, North Shore Long Island Jewish Health System, 270-05 76th Avenue, New Hyde Park, NY 11040, USA; [c] Department of Imaging Sciences, University of Rochester Medical Center, School of Medicine and Dentistry, 601 Elmwood Avenue, Box 648, Rochester, NY 14642, USA
* Corresponding author.
E-mail address: David_Waldman@URMC.Rochester.edu

Ultrasound Clin 8 (2013) 201–212
http://dx.doi.org/10.1016/j.cult.2012.12.014
1556-858X/13/$ – see front matter © 2013 Elsevier Inc. All rights reserved.

ultrasound.theclinics.com

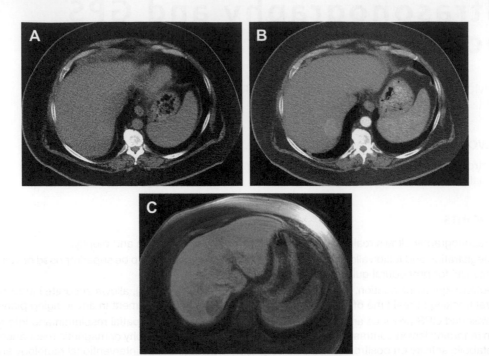

Fig. 1. (*A*) Axial noncontrast computed tomography (CT) demonstrates homogeneous appearance of the liver, without focal lesion visualized. (*B*) Arterial phase postcontrast axial CT makes the enhancing lesion within the posterior right lobe more conspicuous. (*C*) Magnetic resonance (MR) image of abdomen with Eovist in portal venous phase shows lesion washout, suspicious for hepatocellular carcinoma.

guidance is presently another limitation to such procedures. Repositioning of needles and probes costs valuable time, potentially lengthening procedures, and suboptimal placement may worsen the outcome of procedures.[3–5] Accurate placement is made even more difficult by dynamic processes such as breathing and organ movement. Preoperative planning scans may not accurately reflect the true geometries encountered during an interventional procedure.

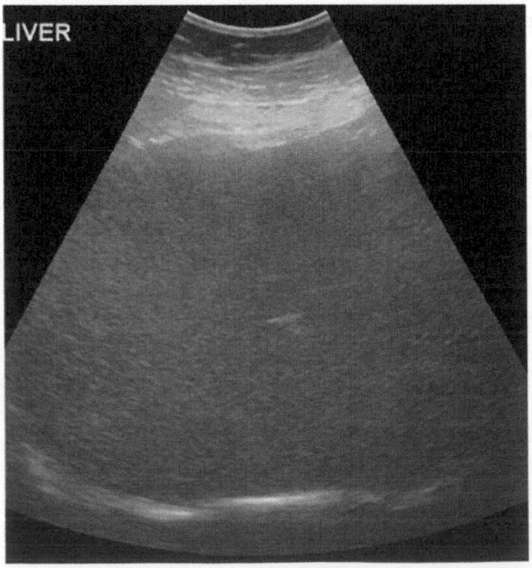

Electromagnetic navigation systems provide a means of simultaneously visualizing and incorporating multiple imaging modalities during guidance while tracking the position and course of a needle or probe in a predetermined imaging volume in real time.[6–8] These systems, akin to global positioning systems (GPS), use the generation of local electromagnetic fields to track interventional radiology devices and ultrasound transducers equipped with miniaturized electromagnetic position sensors. Such systems allow superimposed visualization of real-time ultrasonography with the matched multiplanar reconstruction from a CT, positron emission tomography (PET), or MR imaging examination, granting the benefits of each modality and sidestepping limitations of single-modality guidance. These navigations systems additionally demonstrate the position and course of any needle or probe inserted, even when the device is out of the ultrasound imaging plane.

Understanding the principles, technique, indications, and pitfalls of this technique will become

Fig. 2. Transverse gray-scale sonographic image fails to detect the suspected hepatocellular carcinoma noted in **Fig. 1.**

increasingly important in the clinical practice of interventional radiology, and warrants review.

ULTRASOUND GPS PRINCIPLES

Electromagnetic navigation systems are based on the Biot Savart law, the principle that in the presence of a known magnetic field generator, the magnetic field vector in a given location can be measured in terms of magnitude, direction, length, and the proximity of the current generating the field by a sensor. Knowledge of these variables may be used to determine the position and spatial orientation of the sensor within the field.[9] Miniaturized sensors on the magnitude of needle or probe tips have been developed. This advancement is especially useful, as prior navigation techniques have relied on optical guidance whereby a direct line of site between a camera or infrared sensor and target lesion is required. Electromagnetic navigation, by contrast, allows guidance without direct visualization, almost always necessary in interventional radiology procedures with targets deep within the body.

Electromagnetic navigation systems typically use a small electromagnetic field generator placed in close proximity to the operative field. The field space within which tracking is accurate is relatively small, often on the measure of $50 \times 50 \times 50$ cm, necessitating the close positioning. Most field generators take the form of a small, block-like device mounted from or positioned adjacent to the operative table. This generator creates a small, differential magnetic field into which sensor coils may be placed. These coils detect the rapidly changing magnetic field and, per Faraday's law of electromagnetic induction, elicit a weak electrical current. It is the processing of this current within the magnetic field that allows delineation of sensor, and thus equipment, position within space.

Sensor coils may be placed within or attached to imaging equipment or interventional instruments. Multiple sensors may be tracked simultaneously. At a minimum, sensor coils are attached to the ultrasound transducer being used for real-time guidance, and may be placed within a needle tip, ablation probe, catheter, or guide wire.[10] Sensors placed within interventional instruments allow for localization of these tools within the magnetic field, including with respect to the ultrasound plane being imaged. Needle trajectory is also depicted on the sonogram display, as spatial orientation may be determined in addition to position. The sensor clipped to the ultrasound transducer allows for fusion of the real-time ultrasound plane with a multiplanar reconstructed image from a CT,

PET, or MR data set following the process of coregistration.

Coregistration refers to the process of combining two imaging data sets, one of which represents the real-time ultrasonographic images. At their institution the authors use Volume Navigation on the GE LOGIQ E9 ultrasound system (GE Healthcare, Milwaukee, WI), whereby the registration process is completed manually through the identification of a series of common points on both data sets. Another commonly used commercially available system is the iU22 xMATRIX (Philips Healthcare, Andover, MA), whereby registration may be accomplished by manually matching a series of common anatomic points on both data sets, such as the location and morphology of the hepatic veins. A transformation matrix based on these common data points is applied, which allows display of multiplanar reconstructed CT, MR, or PET images that correspond to the real-time ultrasound plane, and may be displayed adjacent to or superimposed on the image (**Fig. 3**).

Automatic and semiautomatic registration methods have also been described, which allow for more rapid coregistration than the manual process.[11] These semiautomatic registration methods typically use a series of actively tracked, rather than manually registered, fiducial skin markers. Manual registration is more accurate than purely automated techniques at present.

ULTRASOUND GPS PROTOCOL

1. Review preacquired imaging data and plan insertion site for biopsy or ablation probe.
2. Load selected imaging data into ultrasound system for coregistration.
3. Position patient and perform screening ultrasonography to ensure acoustic window.
4. Prepare and drape the patient.
5. Perform manual registration, matching the anatomic position and morphology of similar structures visualized on ultrasonography with those from additional imaging data set.
6. Confirm accuracy of registration.
7. Under ultrasound-guided visualization of target, select insertion site.
8. Insert needle.
9. Track needle and adjust angle based on real-time GPS feedback.
10. (For ablation) Assess treatment response in real time, and adjust as necessary.

Ultrasound-guided procedures using electromagnetic navigation follow a reasonably routine and regimented protocol. A previously described

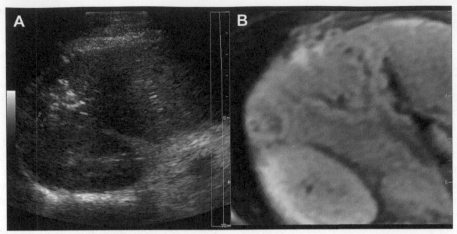

Fig. 3. Coregistered images from real-time ultrasonography (*A*) and historical MR (*B*) displayed in a split-screen format depict an ill-defined hyperechoic lesion on ultrasonography, which correlates with the rim-enhancing posterior right-lobe liver lesion with central washout.

workflow for CT-guided and ultrasound-guided procedures has been published, which requires slight tailoring dependent on the specific case and navigation system available.[8] Imaging data to be used for coregistration should be reviewed, the target evaluated, and an expected insertion site identified (**Fig. 4**). Percutaneous thermoablation cases often require additional planning, with software available that can model predicted zones of adequate heating or cooling and critical structures at risk, and guide the optimal insertion site and number of probes necessary for successful ablation.[3–5] Once preprocedure planning is deemed adequate, the selected imaging data may be loaded into the ultrasound machine to prepare for coregistration (**Fig. 5**). A screening ultrasonogram should be performed to ensure an adequate acoustic window along the planned insertion tract. When positioning and prepping the patient, it is critical to consider the placement and draping of the electromagnetic field generator, which may prove obtrusive given its close proximity to the operating field.[6] The process of registration may then be performed in a manual or automated fashion. At the authors' institution, manual registration is accomplished by matching the morphology of structures within the ultrasound plane with those from CT, MR, or PET imaging. In the liver, for instance, structures such as the hepatic or portal veins often prove useful for this purpose. The accuracy of registration should be confirmed. Under ultrasonographic visualization of the target, the needle may be inserted and tracked in real time to its intended location, making adjustments in angle based on GPS feedback (**Figs. 6 and 7**). Needle location and course can be displayed even if out of plane from the sonographic image, another benefit of this technology (**Fig. 8**).[12]

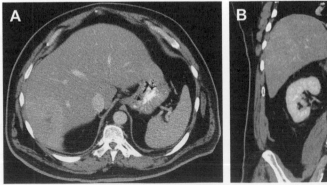

Fig. 4. A 64-year-old man with type 2 diabetes and coronary artery disease presenting with pain in the right upper quadrant. Axial (*A*) and coronal (*B*) postcontrast CT images demonstrate an enhancing, infiltrative lesion within the posterior right lobe of the liver.

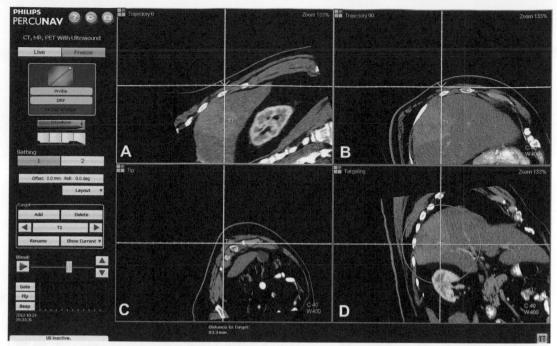

Fig. 5. Preprocedure planning using the PercuNav needle guidance system (Philips Healthcare, Andover, MA). Multiplanar CT reconstructions in the oblique sagittal (*A*) and 90° oblique axial (*B*) planes, depicting the trajectory of the needle toward target (*blue crosshairs*, T1). (*C*) The proposed needle-insertion site is marked (*blue crosshairs*, T1). (*D*) Oblique coronal CT image demonstrates the trajectory of the needle as if looking "down the barrel." The target (*yellow crosshairs*) is surrounded by a green circle, the diameter of which indicates the distance of needle tip to the target.

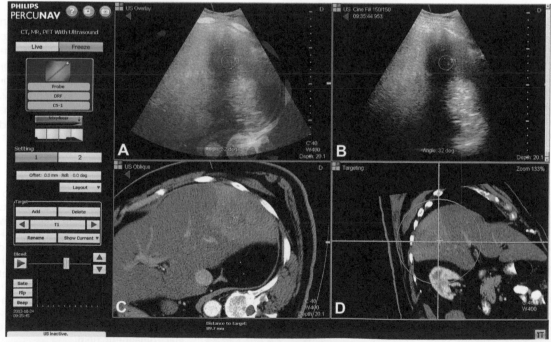

Fig. 6. (*A*) Coregistered real-time ultrasonography image fused with the historical CT, with the needle trajectory (*blue dotted line*) and target (*blue crosshairs*, T1). (*B*) Real-time transverse ultrasonography image demonstrates an ill-defined hypoechoic lesion in the liver, with corresponding oblique transverse historical CT image (*C*). Note the target within the enhancing lesion. (*D*) Oblique coronal CT scan for targeting, with the yellow crosshairs depicting the course of the needle from insertion through target, and the green circle again indicating distance from target.

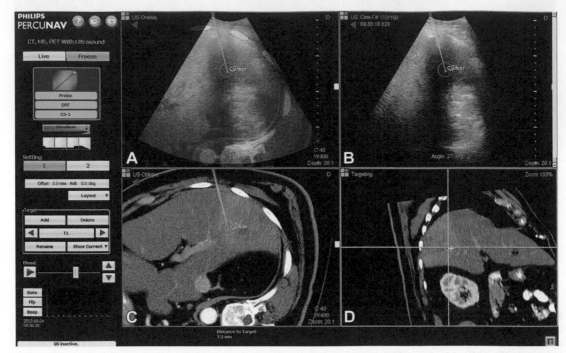

Fig. 7. (*A*) Coregistered real-time sonographic image fused with historical CT. Note the blue line, which depicts the biopsy needle. (*B*) Real-time transverse ultrasonography image with corresponding, coregistered historical CT. (*C, D*) The diameter of the green circle has decreased dramatically, seen on oblique coronal historical CT, indicating that the biopsy needle is near the preselected target.

INDICATIONS

Ultrasound GPS guidance may prove useful in several common interventional radiology procedures. Arterially enhancing lesions, such as hepatomas, which are generally better appreciated on MR or CT, may be biopsied or ablated following fusion of such images to real-time ultrasonography for needle or probe placement. Lesions that present challenging anatomy on biopsy or ablation may be best accessed under electromagnetic guidance. Such technology may also take advantage of coregistration with PET/CT, allowing for the most metabolically active portion of a tumor to be biopsied for improved biopsy sensitivity. Ultrasound–MR imaging fusion has also demonstrated utility in electromagnetically tracked lesion-targeted prostate biopsy.

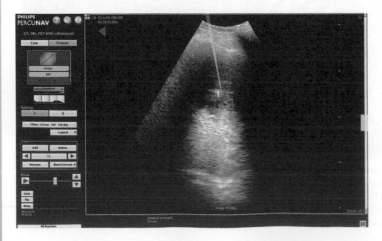

Fig. 8. Gray-scale transverse sonographic image of the liver depicts the echogenic needle tip immediately adjacent to the blue line, which indicates the electromagnetically tracked course of the needle. Note that each terminates at the preselected target lesion. The difference in position represents the total target to registration error, and is the product of registration error and distortion of the electromagnetic field.

CLINICAL APPLICATIONS

An ever increasing number of clinical uses for electromagnetic navigation have been proposed. Extensive research for use in guided bronchoscopy has been published, including a recent publication describing an endobronchial navigation system without a bronchoscope or fiberoptics.[13] Electromagnetic navigation has also been studied in thoracic aortic stent graft deployment and placement of transjugular intrahepatic portosystemic shunt.[14,15] The most common use for ultrasound GPS is in the setting of percutaneous biopsy and ablation.

Percutaneous biopsy and thermal ablation are generally guided by ultrasonography or CT in current practice, as these modalities provide adequate spatial resolution and a means of tracking the biopsy needle during procedure. Many metallic surgical instruments remain impractical for use in MR suites, rendering this modality relatively ineffective. PET offers limited spatial resolution and provides no means for actively tracking a needle to target. CT guidance may be cumbersome, often requiring frequent CT fluoroscopy to assess needle location, as well as repeated repositioning. Moreover, both patient and practitioner receive a significant dose of radiation. Ultrasonography remains an attractive guidance modality, offering real-time feedback without radiation exposure.

ULTRASOUND GPS IN BIOPSY

Ultrasound guidance has traditionally been used for biopsy of soft-tissue lesions, especially within the liver and kidney. Ultrasonography lacks the sensitivity for visualizing some lesions, such as hepatocellular carcinoma, which become more conspicuous following arterial phase-contrast enhancement on CT and MR studies (**Fig. 9**).[16,17] The integration of these modalities by coregistration and fusion for guidance confers the benefits of each, and successful use has been reported in case reports within the literature (**Fig. 10**).[18] Case series have also studied accuracy in the use of ultrasound GPS for biopsy and ablation of liver and renal masses, demonstrating reasonably accurate guidance of needle or probe placement (**Fig. 11**).[19–21]

Ultrasound GPS technology is not limited to the interventional radiology suite, but has also been described in endoscopic ultrasound biopsy of mediastinal lymph nodes.

Lesions considered difficult to be biopsied secondary to complex anatomic positioning may also benefit from the use of electromagnetic

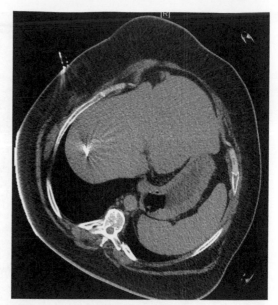

Fig. 9. Attempted CT-guided biopsy of the arterially enhancing lesion from **Fig. 1** resulted in inconclusive results. Lack of lesion visualization contributed to this error.

guidance. Proof of efficacy in further clinical trials is necessary to ensure benefit.

Coregistration of ultrasonographic and PET data may improve the sensitivity of biopsy. The marriage of these modalities ensures biopsy-needle placement in the most metabolically active component of a lesion, which may improve biopsy sensitivity. This technique has proved to be accurate when tested using landmark-based localization, and electromagnetic tracking has proved adequate for biopsy when coregistering real-time ultrasonography with intraprocedural CT, with preacquired ^{18}F-fluorodeoxyglucose PET scan overlaid.[22,23] This method may allow for guided biopsy of subtle, metabolically active lesions not visualized on conventional anatomy-based imaging modalities.

Fused ultrasound-MR electromagnetically guided biopsy of focal prostate lesions has also been demonstrated to be effective.[24] This success offers promise for the guided biopsy or ablation of other lesions best visualized using MR imaging. During prostate biopsy (and biopsy in numerous other organs), motion secondary to respiration, gross patient motion, and pressure exerted by the biopsy device may alter the spatial relationship in comparison with preprocedure imaging. Early attempts to correct for this source of error, using electromagnetic tracking technology following coregistration of MR imaging registered with real-time transrectal ultrasonography for prostate biopsy, offer promise.[25]

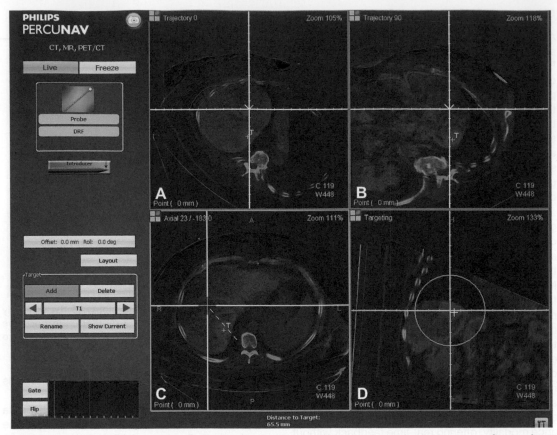

Fig. 10. Successful biopsy was performed using the Philips PercuNav needle guidance system, confirming hepatocellular carcinoma. (*A–C*) Biopsy needle trajectory on coregistered, fused historical MR and CT images in various oblique projections. The yellow crosshairs demonstrate the current position of the needle tip and the blue crosshairs the predetermined target. (*D*) Oblique coronal CT scan for targeting, with the yellow crosshairs depicting the course of the needle from insertion through target, and the green circle again indicating distance from target.

ULTRASOUND GPS IN PERCUTANEOUS ABLATION

Percutaneous thermoablation has become an accepted arm of the treatment paradigm for numerous tumors. Clinical trials have demonstrated efficacy in treating cancers of the liver, kidney, and lung, among others, with thermoablative methods.[26–31] Ablation of such lesions requires careful planning and probe placement.[1,3–5] Numerous ablation probes are often required to treat a single lesion, each with specific dimensions of expected efficacy. Ensuring the success of ablation requires adequate overlap of expected ablation zones from each probe, consideration of collateral damage to healthy and vital organs and structures, and the effects of heat-sink secondary to adjacent blood vessels.[32–34]

Modeling software exists that may aid in planning. This software may apply mathematical or computational models to preablation images to predict zones of adequately heated or cooled tissue to ensure treatment efficacy, and several probe locations may be tested.[3–5,8] The preablation imaging used for planning may be coregistered with the real-time ultrasound-guidance procedure, ensuring more accurate execution of the planned ablation.

Electromagnetic navigation sensors have been incorporated into the radiofrequency ablation (RFA) probe tip, into the coaxial stylet, within the outer cannula of a coaxial sheath, within a guide parallel to the RFA probe, and as an external sensor at the hub of the RFA probe (**Fig. 12**). Each of these has demonstrated accuracy and functionality even during the high temperatures encountered during thermoablation.[35] Furthermore, electromagnetic guidance has been deemed comparable with direct visualization techniques in phantoms, an encouraging sign regarding efficacy.[19]

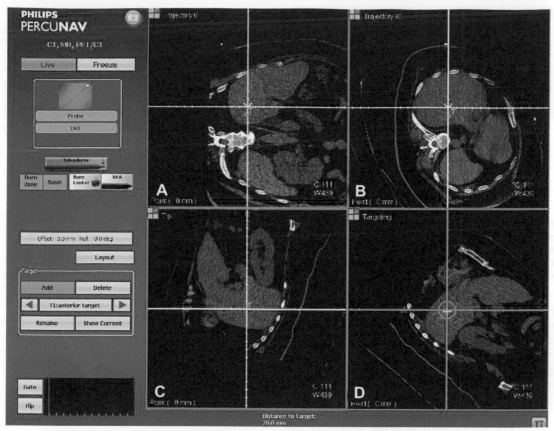

Fig. 11. Philips PercuNav system for radiofrequency ablation of the confirmed hepatocellular carcinoma from Fig. 10. (*A–C*) Needle trajectory in various imaging planes using the historical CT. Yellow crosshairs demonstrate the position of the trocar tip and blue crosshairs show the preselected target. (*D*) Oblique coronal image for targeting. The green circle, with small diameter, confirms that the depth of the needle tip is approaching the intended target.

Although ultrasonography offers real-time guidance, its use as an image-guidance technique for guided ablation has been limited. The ice ball produced during cryoablation may cause posterior acoustic shadowing on conventional sonography,[36] and gas bubbles formed as a result of heat production during microwave or RFA may yield "gassing out" of the treatment region (**Fig. 13**).[37,38] Fusion of real-time ultrasound guidance with the spatial resolution and contrast-enhanced capabilities of CT or MR, or knowledge of metabolic activity garnered from

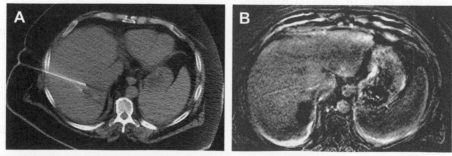

Fig. 12. (*A*) Axial CT confirms accurate placement of trocars placed for radiofrequency ablation, guided by the Philips PercuNav system. (*B*) Subtraction axial MR image post Eovist 6 months after treatment confirms successful radiofrequency ablation of the hepatocellular carcinoma.

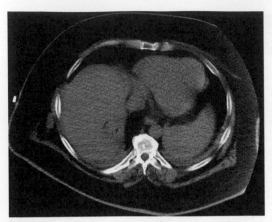

Fig. 13. Axial CT immediately following electromagnetic-guided radiofrequency ablation demonstrates gas within the ablation cavity, which causes gassing out when ultrasound is used for ablation guidance.

PET, allows for intraprocedural adjustment to ensure adequate lesion coverage despite insufficient guidance from ultrasound alone.

PITFALLS OF ULTRASOUND GPS

Tracking error
1. Registration error: difference between 2 like points from separate data sets following coregistration
2. Distortion of magnetic field, causing errors in tracking of sensors

Limited functional volume

Obtrusive equipment

Time-consuming process

Though offering substantial promise, electromagnetic navigation is not without flaws. Electromagnetic guidance relies on several complex technologies working in concert to ensure success. Each of these technologies provides a potential source of procedural error.

Error within the system may arise from failure of registration and failure of tracking following registration. Registration error, the difference between how well 2 like points match between 2 coregistered data sets, is desired to be less than 2 mm.[8,11] Most manual registration methods can attain such accuracy; with fully automatic registration methods coming close.[11] Distortion of the generated electromagnetic field may lead to inaccurate localization of sensors within the system. Such distortion may arise from ferromagnetic objects within the field or vicinity, and may contribute to additional tracking errors. Commonly encountered sources of distortion in the interventional radiology suite include the

C-arm or CT scanner. The total target to registration error, or difference between real and virtual needle positions, amounts to an average of 3 to 5 mm in systems tested within the clinical environment.[6,11] Though small, in select cases this error may result in sufficient inaccuracy to worsen outcomes.

The limited functional volume of most commercially available electromagnetic navigation systems also hampers its utility. Functional volume defines the volume of space within which the introduced magnetic field is capable of garnering a measurable induced voltage from an electromagnetic sensor, thus discerning position. Functional volume presently measures approximately $50 \times 50 \times 50$ cm; this demands close placement of the electromagnetic field generator, which may prove obtrusive during procedures.

The effect on procedure time of using electromagnetic navigation has yet to be fully evaluated. In the authors' experience, the additional time required for loading preacquired studies, attaining adequate registration, and arranging and draping the electromagnetic field generator offset any theoretical gains from more direct guidance and fewer needle-angle adjustments. This balance may improve if such devices are more seamlessly incorporated into ultrasound machines, and if automatic registration is deemed accurate enough for guidance. Further work limiting distortion of the electromagnetic field, expanding functional volume, and improving accuracy could also result in more mainstream acceptance of electromagnetic navigation.

SUMMARY

Ultrasonography offers real-time guidance for many procedures within interventional radiology, including percutaneous ablation and biopsy. As technology evolves, incorporating ultrasound GPS promises to expand this role and improve outcomes in such procedures.

VIDEOS

Videos related to this article can be found online at http://dx.doi.org/10.1016/j.cult.2012.12.014.

REFERENCES

1. Goldberg SN, Grassi CJ, Cardella JF, et al. Image-guided tumor ablation: standardization of terminology and reporting criteria. Radiology 2005;235:728–39.
2. Allen BC, Remer EM. Percutaneous cryoablation of renal tumors: patient selection, technique, and postprocedural imaging. RadioGraphics 2010;30:887–900.

3. Dodd GD, Frank MS, Aribandi M, et al. Radiofrequency thermal ablation: computer analysis of the size of thermal injury created by overlapping ablations. AJR Am J Roentgenol 2001;177(4):777–92.

4. Chen CR, Miga MI, Galloway RI. "Optimizing needle placement in treatment planning of radiofrequency ablation". Proc. SPIE;614:614124-1. Available at: http://dx.doi.org/10.1117/12.654983. Accessed July 5, 2012.

5. Banovac F, Abeledo H, Campos-Nanez E, et al. An image-guided system for optimized volumetric treatment planning and execution for radiofrequency ablation of liver tumors. Int J Comput Assist Radiol Surg 2007;2(Suppl 1):S146–51.

6. Wilson E, Yaniv Z, Lindisch D, et al. Electromagnetic tracking in the clinical environment. Med Phys 2009; 36(3):876–92.

7. Wood BJ, Zhang H, Durrani A, et al. Navigation with electromagnetic tracking for interventional radiology procedures: a feasibility study. J Vasc Interv Radiol 2005;16:493–505.

8. Wood BJ, Kruecker J, Abi-Jaoudeh N, et al. Navigation systems for ablation. J Vasc Interv Radiol 2010; 21:S256–63.

9. Baszynski M, Moron Z, Tewel N. Electromagnetic navigation in medicine- basic issues, advantages and shortcomings, prospects for improvement. J Phys 2010. Conf Series 238 012056. Available at: http://dx/doi.org/10.1088/1742-6596/238/1/0/012056. Accessed June 25, 2012.

10. Locklin J, Kruecker J, Xu S, et al. Abstract no. 156. Clinical trial for "smart" interventional devices using an image navigation fusion system. J Vasc Interv Radiol 2008;19:S60.

11. Krucker J, Xu S, Glossop N, et al. Electromagnetic tracking for thermal ablation and biopsy guidance: clinical evaluation of spatial accuracy. J Vasc Interv Radiol 2007;18:1141–50.

12. Wallace MJ, Gupta S, Hicks ME. Out-of-plane computed-tomography-guided biopsy using a magnetic-field-based navigation system. Cardiovasc Intervent Radiol 2006;29:108–13.

13. Sharma K, Xu S, Glossop N, et al. Abstract no. 310. Steerable endobronchial navigation without a bronchoscope or fiberoptics. J Vasc Interv Radiol 2008; 19:S114–5.

14. Abi-Jaoudeh N, Dake MD, Prichard WF, et al. Abstract no. 245. Electromagnetic tracking navigation for thoracic aortic stent graft deployment. J Vasc Interv Radiol 2009;20:S94.

15. Levy EB, Zhang H, Lindisch D, et al. Electromagnetic tracking-guided percutaneous intrahepatic portosystemic shunt creation in a swine model. J Vasc Interv Radiol 2007;18:303–7.

16. Yu NC, Chaudhari V, Raman SS, et al. CT and MRI improve detection of hepatocellular carcinoma, compared with ultrasound alone, in patients with cirrhosis. Clin Gastroenterol Hepatol 2011;9:161–7.

17. Teefey SA, Hildebolt CC, Dehdashti F, et al. Detection of primary hepatic malignancy in liver transplant candidates: prospective comparison of CT, MR imaging, US, and PET. Radiology 2003;226: 533–42.

18. Buckner CA, Venkatesan A, Locklin JK, et al. Real-time sonography with electromagnetic tracking navigation for biopsy of a hepatic neoplasm seen only on arterial phase computed tomography. J Ultrasound Med 2011;30:253–6.

19. Saxena V, Beck A, Kapoor A, et al. Abstract no. 117. Accuracy of RFA probe insertions using camera-on-needle versus electromagnetic tracking. J Vasc Interv Radiol 2010;21:S46.

20. Amalou H, Abi-Jaoudeh N, Venkatesen A, et al. Abstract no. 71. Fusion guided biopsy or ablation: clinical trial update in 461 patients. J Vasc Interv Radiol 2012;23:S32.

21. Krucker J, Xu S, Venkatesan A, et al. Clinical utility of real-time fusion guidance for biopsy and ablation. J Vasc Interv Radiol 2011;22:515–24.

22. Kadoury S, Wood BJ, Venkatesan A, et al. Accuracy assessment of an automatic image-based PET/CT registration for ultrasound-guided biopsies and ablations. Proc SPIE 2011;7964:79642P. Available at: http://dx.doi.org/10.1117/12.878067. Accessed July 30, 2012.

23. Venkatesan A, Kadoury S, Abi-Jaoudeh N, et al. Real-time FDG PET guidance during biopsies and radiofrequency ablation using multimodality fusion with electromagnetic navigation. Radiology 2011; 260(3):848–56.

24. Venkatesan A, Krucker J, Xu S, et al. Abstract no. 155. Early clinical experience with real time ultrasound MRI fusion-guided prostate biopsies. J Vasc Interv Radiol 2008;19:S59–60.

25. Xu S, Kruecker J, Turkbey B, et al. Evaluation of motion correction in fused MRI/TRUS guided prostate biopsy. J Vasc Interv Radiol 2009;20: S137–8.

26. Howard JH, Tzeng CW, Smith JK, et al. Radiofrequency ablation for unresectable tumors of the liver. Am Surg 2008;74(7):594–600 [discussion: 600–1].

27. Lencioni R, Cioni D, Crocetti L, et al. Early-stage hepatocellular carcinoma in patients with cirrhosis: long-term results of percutaneous image-guided radiofrequency ablation. Radiology 2005;234: 961–7.

28. Zagoria RJ, Pettus JA, Rogers M, et al. Long-term outcomes after percutaneous radiofrequency ablation for renal cell carcinoma. Urology 2011;77: 1393–7.

29. Davol PE, Fulmer BR, Rukstalis DB. Long-term results of cryoablation for renal cancer and complex renal masses. Urology 2006;68(Suppl 1A):2–6.

30. Simon CJ, Dupuy DE, DiPetrillo TA, et al. Pulmonary radiofrequency ablation: long-term safety and efficacy in 153 patients. Radiology 2007;243: 268–75.

31. Vogl TJ, Naguib NN, Gruber-Rouh T, et al. Microwave ablation therapy: clinical utility in treatment of pulmonary metastases. Radiology 2011;261: 643–51.

32. Goldber SN, Han PF, Hapera EP, et al. Radiofrequency tissue ablation: effect of pharmacologic modulation of blood flow on coagulation diameter. Radiology 1998;209:762–7.

33. Lu DS, Raman SS, Limanond P, et al. Influence of large peritumoral vessels on outcome of radiofrequency ablations of liver tumors. J Vasc Interv Radiol 2003;14:1267–74.

34. Rieder C, Schwier M, Weinhusen A, et al. Visualization of risk structures for interactive planning for image guided radiofrequency ablation of liver tumors. Proc SPIE 2009;7261:726134-1. Available at: http://dx.doi.org/10.1117/12.813729. Accessed August 5, 2012.

35. Razjouyan F, Kapoor A, Glossop N, et al. A comparison of methods for tracking RFA probes and sensitivity to RF field and temperature. J Vasc Interv Radiol J Vasc Inter Radiol 2010;21:S46–7.

36. Hinshaw JL, Shadid AM, Nakada SY, et al. Comparison of percutaneous and laparoscopic cryoablation for treatment of solid renal masses. Am J Roentgenol 2008;191:1159–68.

37. Goldber SN, Gazelle GS, Solbiati L, et al. Ablation of liver tumors using percutaneous RF therapy. Am J Roentgenol 1998;170:1023–8.

38. Wood BJ, Locklin JK, Viswanathan A, et al. Techniques for guidance of radiofrequency ablation in the multimodality interventional suite of the future. J Vasc Interv Radiol 2007;18 (1 Pt 1):9–24.

High-intensity Focused Ultrasound

George A. Holland, MD[a,†], Oleg Mironov, MD[a],
Jean-Francois Aubry, PhD[b,c],
Arik Hananel, MD, MBA, BsCS[d,e], Jeremy B. Duda, MD[a,*]

KEYWORDS

- Magnetic resonance-guided focused ultrasound surgery • High-intensity focused ultrasound
- Therapy • Thermal ablation • Drug therapy • Uterine fibroid

KEY POINTS

- Focused ultrasound, also known as high-intensity focused ultrasound, uses an ultrasound beam generated from a large transducer or array of transducers, which is focused to a small focal point (similar to a magnifying glass) to exert an effect in deep tissue, with the intent of sparing surrounding tissues from the effect.
- FUS has many current and potential medical applications ranging from creating transient cellular membrane permeability (for drug delivery, modification of blood-brain barrier to improve drug efficacy, or potential aid in genetic therapy) to thermal heating for tumor and diseased tissue ablation.
- To perform these therapies, it is necessary to identify the abnormal tissue needing treatment and surrounding tissues that need to be spared.
- Magnetic resonance imaging is currently the best imaging technique for this purpose.
- Magnetic resonance imaging has the best tissue contrast and can determine temperature changes from 2°C to 3°C at 1 T to 1°C at 3 T.

HISTORY

The piezoelectric effect was discovered in the early 1900s. Woods and Lumis performed initial work of investigating high-intensity ultrasound in animals in 1927. In 1935 Gruetzmacher published the first report on focusing ultrasound, using a piezoelectric transducer with a concave surface. From 1942 to 1955, both Lynn and colleagues[1] and the Fry brothers (Francis and William) demonstrated deep tissue damage in bovine liver and cat brain, respectively, without surrounding effects.[2]

Ablation of malignant tissues was first proposed by Burov in 1956 with subsequent research performed by Fry and coworkers.[3] Ferenc Jolesz and his colleagues[4–7] at the Brigham and Women's Hospital in Boston, along with InSightec (Haifa, Israel), have spearheaded research and development in magnetic resonance (MR)-guided focused ultrasound (FUS) applications in the body and brain. This work has resulted in the US Food and Drug Administration (FDA) approval of an MR-guided FUS system manufactured by

[a] Department of Imaging Sciences, University of Rochester Medical Center, 601 Elmwood Avenue, Box 648, Rochester, NY 14642, USA; [b] Department of Neurosurgery, Radiation Oncology, The University of Virginia School of Medicine, Charlottesville, VA 22903; [c] Institut Langevin, ESPCI, 10, rue Vauquelin, 75005 Paris, France; [d] Department of Radiation Oncology, The University of Virginia School of Medicine, Charlottesville, VA 22908, USA; [e] Focused Ultrasound Surgery Foundation, 1230 Cedars Court, Suite F, Charlottesville, VA 22903, USA
[†] Deceased. With deep sadness the co-authors would like to acknowledge Dr George A. Holland's unexpected and tragic death which occurred during the publication of this article. Dr Holland touched all of our lives with his outsized generosity, bombastic personality and his infectious sense of humor. He was a fearless, tireless physician, a brilliant teacher and dedicated mentor. We dedicate this article to him.
* Corresponding author.
E-mail address: jeremy_duda@urmc.rochester.edu

Ultrasound Clin 8 (2013) 213–226
http://dx.doi.org/10.1016/j.cult.2012.12.015
1556-858X/13/$ – see front matter © 2013 Elsevier Inc. All rights reserved.

InSightec. Philips (Philips Healthcare, Andover MA) now has an MR-guided high-intensity focused ultrasound (HIFU) under FDA trials in the United States and in use in Europe.

PHYSICS
Ultrasound

When ultrasound (US) vibrations traverse tissue, they are attenuated by soft tissues by a factor of approximately 0.3 dB/cm for a 1-MHz signal. Signal energy that is lost is converted to heat given by the expression

$$Q = \frac{\alpha p^2}{\rho c}$$

where Q is the heat generated per unit volume, α is absorption coefficient, which increases with frequency, p is the pressure amplitude, ρ is density, and c is the speed of sound in tissue. The distribution of heat within a tissue can then be modeled using Pennes' bioheat equation, which takes into account tissue perfusion, the specific heat of the tissue and blood, and the thermal conductivity of tissue.[8]

To damage specific diseased structures and to leave healthy tissue intact, the US beam is focused on a small area. By doing so, energy is deposited disproportionately on a specific site, analogous to focusing light with a magnifying glass to create a hotspot. With FUS, a phased array of US elements electronically steers the beam to its target.

The focal point of a focused beam is ellipsoid with dimensions given by the equation:

$$\Delta x = \lambda \frac{F}{D} \qquad \Delta z = 7 \times \lambda \left(\frac{F}{D}\right)^2$$

where x represents the short-axis diameter, z is the long axis diameter (both defined as the edges of one-half of the peak intensity), D is the transducer aperture, F is the focal distance, and λ is the wavelength. As can be seen from this equation, use of smaller US windows such as between ribs or ablation of deeper tissues lengthens the focal spot, in a geometric manner. The tightest focal spot is achieved by treating shallower tissues and using the largest possible acoustic window. The larger the transducer aperture is relative to the focal distance (ie, a lower f_{number}), the better the focus quality is.

$$f_{number} = \frac{F}{D}$$

In current clinical devices, $f_{numbers}$ typically range from 0.5 to 1.5. For a given f_{number}, using a higher transmit frequency results in a tighter focus because of the shorter wavelength (as seen in the first equation). Transmitted frequencies for HIFU typically range from 0.2 MHz to 4 MHz. High frequencies provide a better f_{number} and will spare tissues in the far field, but may cause excessive heating in the near field. Transmitting with a low frequency will spare the near field tissues, have better penetration into deeper structures, but will compromise the f_{number} and may result in excessive heating in the far field (**Fig. 1**).

Tissue damage caused by FUS is primarily caused by local heating, which is predictable and can be monitored during the procedure. Another effect that can occur during sonication is called cavitation. Cavitation, which tends to occur at high intensities, is caused by formation of microbubbles within the tissue. These microbubbles absorb US energy efficiently and collapse, causing rapid tissue damage as shockwaves and high-speed liquid jets are released, at very high temperatures and pressures, leading to mechanical disruption of tissue. An increase in acoustic intensity can transform

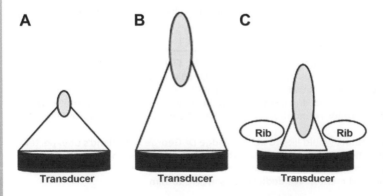

A   **B**   **C**

Rib   Rib

Transducer   Transducer   Transducer

Fig. 1. Effect of differences in f_{number} or beam path on ablation zones. Ellipses represent the areas of energy deposition, with the edges receiving one-fourth of the energy at the center of the focus. (*A*) Shallow tissue with a large window; this is the optimal configuration because the ablation zone is well focused with minimal effect on the far and near fields. (*B*) Deep tissue with a large US window. Here the unfavorable f_{number} causes greater effect on the far and near fields manifested as a wider area of energy deposition. (*C*) Small US window. Again an unfavorable f_{number} causes a greater effect in the far and near fields.

a stable cavitation to an inertial or transient cavitation. Inertial cavitation, or histotripsy, is characterized by imploding bubbles, which are powerful enough to liquefy the tissue. Cavitation cannot be predicted or monitored at this time and is typically avoided so as not to cause unintended injury. Current work aims to produce accurate models of this phenomenon in the hopes of producing therapeutic applications in FUS.[9,10]

Changes in the cellular architecture induced by tissue cavitation and heating can alter acoustic interfaces, which can distort, reflect, or refract the US beam along its path to the target. If treatment parameters are held constant, the focal point can change location and intensity because of this interference. Energy deposition by the US beam may then be redirected to nontarget sites during the course of a treatment, not only creating the potential for complications but also decreasing the effectiveness of the treatment on the target. Monitoring with a wide field-of-view such as with MR imaging may allow adjustments to the beam to ensure a safe and effective procedure.

One potential complication noted by investigators during development of FUS arose during treatment of large fields: after the end of a sonication, continued heating was detected in areas near the ablated tissue. Initially a cool-down time between successive sonications was incorporated into the treatments to reduce heating and prevent unintentional injuries. Recent articles have investigated the use of interleaved and spiral patterns of sonication to allow shorter cool down and therefore shorter treatments.[11,12]

Monitoring

Monitoring of FUS therapy can be performed with MR imaging, which provides 3-dimensional anatomic details and allows accurate targeting of the US beam. Nearly real-time, noninvasive thermometry of treated tissue is achievable based on the temperature dependence of MR signals.

Several methods of monitoring with MR imaging have been evaluated, with advantages and disadvantages. Thus far, the best results have been achieved by measuring the proton resonance frequency shift (PRF), also known as the Larmor frequency. The resonant frequency of any given proton is dependent on its local magnetic field. This local magnetic field is a function of the external magnetic field and the shielding, also called the screening constant.

$$B_{loc} = B_0 - B_0 s = (1 - s)B_0$$

where B_{loc} is the local magnetic field, B_0 is the field established by the main magnet, and s is the screening constant. The resonant frequency then takes on the form of

$$\omega = \gamma B_0(1 - s)$$

where ω is the Larmor frequency and γ is the gyromagnetic ratio.

The shielding constant is determined by the chemical bonds surrounding a proton. Water efficiently screens protons; however, when hydrogen bonding occurs such as in liquid water, the screening is decreased. As temperature increases, water molecules break their hydrogen bonds more often, allowing the proton to spend more time being screened. This screening causes an inverse, linear relationship between temperature and the PRF and allows a relatively accurate evaluation of the latter in a range of $-15°C$ to $100°C$.

This effect can be measured with spectroscopy or with a gradient echo sequence. Spectroscopy permits determination of the absolute temperature, but has poor temporal and spatial resolution. Therefore, the preferred method is phase change comparison using gradient echo sequence of pre-ablation and postablation images, which only permits measurement of temperature relative to other tissues. The temperature measurements can also be performed more rapidly with echoplanar techniques. However, echoplanar methods are more sensitive to susceptibility artifacts that occur near gas, calcium, and metal.

A significant limitation of PRF monitoring is that water protons in fat have a very weak relationship to temperature. Because these protons can form fewer hydrogen bonds, thermometry is more difficult in fat-containing tissues such as the breast. The problem can be overcome with T1 imaging. T1-weighted imaging is also sensitive to temperature. However, the relationship to temperature varies in different tissues and can become nonlinear at temperatures as low as $43°C$. These constraints make its use somewhat limited.[13]

Contrast agents that raise the signal-to-noise ratio of PRF have been developed; however, their utility is somewhat limited given the lengths of FUS treatments (**Figs. 2–5**).

CLINICAL APPLICATIONS FOR MR-GUIDED FUS THERAPY

Currently MR-guided FUS is performed using an integrated system, and several preparatory steps are necessary to optimize therapy. To maximize transmission of US energy into the body, the patient's skin must be adequately prepared by removing hair and cleaning the contact area with alcohol. For uterine fibroids, a pelvic gel pad, US

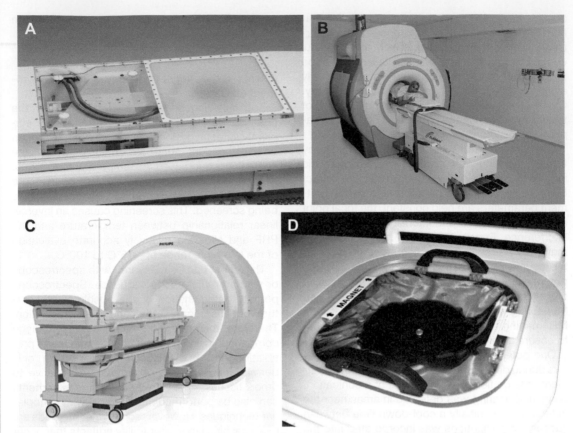

Fig. 2. (*A, B*) (*left*) Focused ultrasound transducer in a bath of water located in the MR table. The phased array is located on a robotic arm. The array has 208 elements. (*right*) Complete MR-guided FUS system with patient on table in a General Electric MR scanner. This system has been approved for clinical use for the treatment of uterine fibroids in the United States. (*C*) Combined Philips MR scanner. (*D*) HIFU transducer embedded in the table. This system is currently undergoing trials for FDA approval. (*D*) Close up of embedded transducer. ([*A, B*] *Courtesy of* InSightec, Inc, Tirat Carmel, Israel; with permission; [*C*] *Courtesy of* Philips, Andover, MA; with permission.)

gel, and degassed water are used to assure acoustic coupling.

Pelvic Organs (Uterus and Prostate)

Uterine fibroids and adenomyomas

The first FDA-approved indication for FUS treatment is for symptomatic uterine fibroids. According to the Focused Ultrasound Foundation, more than 10,000 patients worldwide have undergone treatment with MR-guided FUS to date. Uterine fibroids occur in greater than 50% of women[14] and are the leading cause of hysterectomy in the United States.[15] Symptomatic onset usually occurs in the premenopausal period, with menorrhagia, dysmenorrhea, urinary frequency, nocturia, and pelvic pain/pressure.[16–19]

A preprocedure MR image should be obtained to evaluate the sizes and locations of the fibroids. Most clinical studies have generally described treatments of 2-cm to 12-cm fibroids. With advances in technology and increased speed, the size of fibroids that can be treated with magnetic resonance-guided focused ultrasound surgery (MRgFUS) may increase.

The MR image should also be reviewed for potential areas of problem such as abdominal wall scars or metallic foreign bodies because these will interfere with or alter the treatment. In additional, care should be taken to assess whether any bowel is in the way of the beam. The relative position of the uterus can be adjusted to allow a clear beam path by filling/emptying the bladder to avoid bowel or scar. The rectum can also be filled with water or US gel if the fibroid is too far from the transducer.

Once the initial adjustments have been performed, the procedure can begin. A test sonication is performed for calibration, followed by treatment sonications. The procedure is monitored by a radiologist, who may adjust treatment parameters based on MR imaging findings to ensure adequate beam is focusing and to prevent nontarget heating. Because the focal area is relatively small, on the

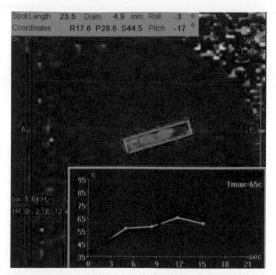

Fig. 3. Phase contrast image with time-temperature plot. MR image permits real-time temperature monitoring (originally every 3 seconds, but now every 0.3 seconds on using echoplanar techniques at 1.5 T, which can be even faster at 3 T). The green area in the image denotes tissue that has reached therapeutic temperature for an adequate period of time to create an ablation. Magnitude images are also available to monitor the anatomy being treated. The graph denotes the temperature on the x-axis in degrees Centigrade over a 15-second period with time on the y-axis in seconds.

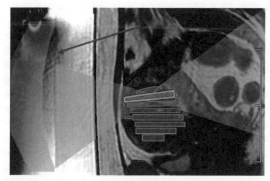

Fig. 4. Beam shaping. Sagittal T2-weighted scan reveals a uterine fibroid. The blue parabolic structure on the left represents the phased array. The red arrow points to the transducer array. The bright hyperintense area is the water in which the array is located. There is a Mylar layer between the patient and a gel pad on which the patient lies. The blue triangle on the left of the image near the transducer is the near field. The blue triangle on the right of the image on the posterior aspect of the patient is the far field. The green boxes are the planned spots to be treated. The size, orientation, and parameters used on each spot can be manipulated individually to avoid or decrease the risk to surrounding structures. Philips uses a continuously moving spiral trajectory.

order of 2 × 1 × 1 cm, overlapping sonications are performed for most lesions. The size of the ablation zone can be increased to 4 cm in length. Philips uses a continuous spiral technique. During early work, FUS treatments could last up to 3 hours, but over the last few years, the average length of the procedure has decreased to approximately 1 to 3 hours. For larger fibroids, the patient may need more than 1 treatment. Following completion of the treatment, a contrast-enhanced MR should be performed to assess the treated lesion and evaluate for complications. The nonenhancing area corresponding to treated tumor may differ from the monitoring images because of limitations in MR thermometry.

The treatment is well tolerated and requires conscious sedation. A compression stocking should be worn during the procedure to prevent deep venous thrombosis. The recovery time usually lasts a few hours to 1 day. Common complications of this technique include minor skin burns and subcutaneous and muscular edema, all of which tend to be self-limited and can be prevented by attention to skin preparation, assessment for scars, and limiting the total treatment time. Transient nerve injury has been reported as a result of bone heating in 3 cases, according to InSightec. It should be noted that these cases occurred before software features that calculate heating of bone at or near the nerves. Clearance of 2 cm from the posterior aspect of the treatment area to the sacrum is recommended to minimize risk. Two cases of bowel injury have also been reported by InSightec, a complication that can be prevented by correct identification of the bowel on the pretreatment MR image as well as with active monitoring of the procedure.[20]

Extensive clinical evaluation has led to the approval of MRgFUS by the FDA for fibroid ablation. Although early studies showed small reductions in the size of fibroids and relatively low rates of symptom resolution, these studies were limited by small treatment volumes because of initial concerns about safety. A more recent study aimed at the treatment of a larger fibroid volume was conducted with 130 patients and 12 months of follow-up, finding a near 90% reduction of symptoms that persisted at 12 months.[21]

Some studies have examined after procedure morbidity such as fertility after ablation. The largest study to date describes 51 women who became pregnant after the procedure, with 41% live births, 28% spontaneous abortions, 11% elective termination, and 20% ongoing pregnancy beyond 20 weeks.[22]

Focal adenomyomas have also been successfully treated with MR-guided FUS (**Figs. 6** and **7**).[23,24]

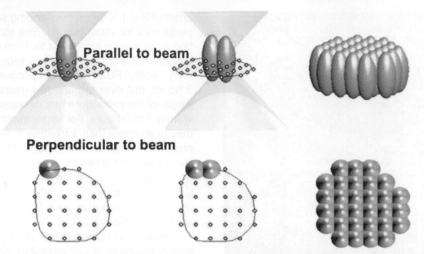

Fig. 5. Initially MRgFUS used contiguous spots to fill in the area to be treated, producing overlapping near and far fields. The procedure requires up to 90 seconds of cooling time between each treatment to prevent injury to non-targeted tissue surrounding these areas. Development of the InSightec machine has reduced nontarget ablation using a technique known as "interleaving," using a computer-generated algorithm that separates target zones.

Prostate

One of every 6 men will develop prostate cancer, and most of these will present at an early, confined stage, due in part to routine surveillance with

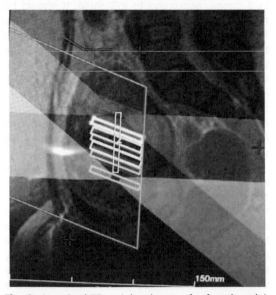

Fig. 6. A sagittal T2-weighted scan of a female pelvis with a uterine fibroid showing application of the interleaved sonication method. The beam paths are denoted in green and blue. Note that spaces between the beam paths and the spots are separated with less overlap of near and far fields. The decreasing of the overlap decreases cooling time, which allows faster treatment. The purple line is placed by the treating physician to demarcate the area of bowel and the red crosses are placed to identify bony structures that need to be used by the system to insure that the beams do not injure these structures.

laboratory markers and heightened clinical awareness.[25,26] Conventional treatment of low-risk lesions is varied and controversial, because patients may elect to have radical prostatectomy or watchful waiting, weighing the rate of morbidity of surgery in their decision.[27,28] HIFU has enormous potential in the treatment of localized prostate tumors, which offers another potential conservative route of therapy. In addition, HIFU may also have a role as a salvage or combination therapy such as in drug delivery.[29]

Regional anatomy of the pelvis makes the technical application of HIFU for prostate disease unique. The prostate gland can be accessed via a transurethral or transrectal approach, allowing a good sonographic window for treatment; the latter technique has enabled the success of other US-guided procedures in the prostate.[30,31] MR imaging of the pelvis is particularly successful and has been shown to demonstrate superior anatomy of the prostate gland, especially at 3.0 T, which can delineate critical nerve bundles as well as tumor margins. However, HIFU for the prostate, similar to the treatment of uterine fibroids, must balance delivery of adequate dose for tumor destruction with the target's proximity to bowel and bladder in the near field, monitoring of the sacrum and nerve roots in the far field, as well as local complications.[32]

Monitoring and guidance is critical for the clinical success of HIFU for the prostate. Nearly all of the clinical research has been performed in Europe and Asia[33] using 2 commercially available US-guided units, and although its use is approved in various countries, it is widely considered an

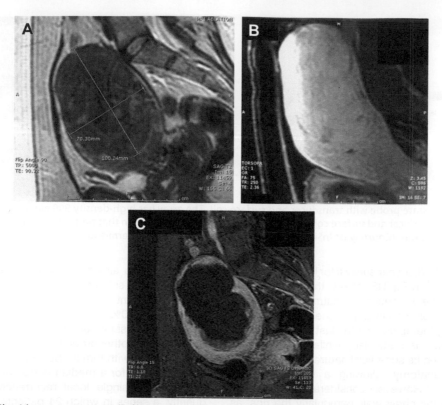

Fig. 7. (*A*) Fibroid pretreatment T2 (*left*). (*B*) T1 with contrast (*right*). (*C*) Fibroid after treatment T1 with contrast (*right*) shows no enhancement, indicating nonviable tissue from the same patient.

experimental treatment.[34] One recent systematic review of 20 case series found favorable overall rates of biochemical and pathologic remission, and promising overall survival, but graded the overall evidence as very low given the severe limitations of these studies.[33] A recent prospective study targeting focal tumors found promising tumor control and low genitourinary-related side effects. No randomized controlled trials have been performed to date.

MR imaging has significant advantages over US guidance; however, technology for its use is still in development, primarily in feasibility studies. For instance, a Canadian group successfully performed MRgFUS treatments on 8 subjects with low-risk disease using a transurethral probe,[30] and other groups are investigating a transrectal probe. MRgFUS is in its infancy, as proof of feasibility and efficacy remains the goal of current work (**Fig. 8**).

Musculoskeletal and Soft Tissue Applications

Bone

FUS has been investigated for the palliative treatment of bone metastasis. To date, the Exablate

system has gained regulatory approval in Europe for this indication and has been FDA approved in 2012.

The principles of treatment are similar to fibroids. Bone absorbs US energy more efficiently than fibroids or other soft tissues, Which permits the use of a lower energy US beam and larger focal spots. A small trial of 32 patients with symptomatic bone metastases demonstrated pain relief in 72% of patients who completed the treatment and were still alive on follow-up. No significant adverse events were reported.[35] Treatment of primary bone tumors has also been attempted. Complications included first-degree skin burns (20%), 1 third-degree skin burn and nerve damage (12%) (**Fig. 9**).[36]

Breast

Breast cancer affects 1 in 8 women, 60% of whom will present with a tumor confined to the primary site.[37]

Although modified radical mastectomy was once the mainstay of treatment of localized breast cancer, large-scale studies have proven the effectiveness of local excision combined with chemotherapy and radiation.[38,39] Indeed, between

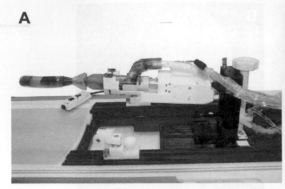 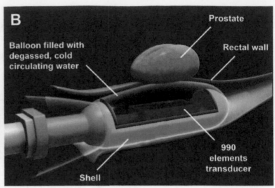

Fig. 8. (*A*) Prostate probe with transducer and surface coil. The array has high-density 990 elements. (*B*) A depiction of the transducer and surface coil. This endocavitary probe has a balloon that permits circulating cool fluid to protect the rectum. (*Courtesy of* InSightec, Inc, Tirat Carmel, Israel; with permission.)

2005 and 2008, 5-year survival for localized tumors was 98.4%. MRgFUS offers the potential for a noninvasive yet definitive treatment of localized breast cancer, continuing in the arc of breast-conserving therapies over the last several years.

The breast is particularly well-suited for HIFU therapy given its superficial nature and lack of obstructing anatomy, allowing a wide treatment window.[32,40] However, consideration of far-field effects on the chest wall, particularly the ribs, as well as reflection by the air-filled lungs and structures in the mediastinum must be included in treatment planning.

Because of concerns about near and far-field monitoring, MR-guided FUS systems have been developed and tested, for instance, the FUS apparatus by InSightec.[41,42] In this apparatus, the breast is lowered into an MR image surface coil, similar to conventional breast MR machines, which fits into a tub containing the transducer and a cooling bath. Intravenous contrast is administered and the postcontrast images are used for treatment planning.

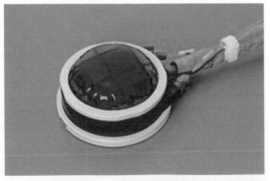

Fig. 9. Conformal transducer for bone treatment. The array has 1000 elements. (*Courtesy of* InSightec, Inc, Tirat Carmel, Israel; with permission.)

Initial studies aimed at preoperative treatment with HIFU and subsequent pathologic evaluation of the treatment zone for residual tumor found that between 90% and 100% of the tumor volume could be successfully ablated[40] in a small group of 25 patients. Another group followed a small cohort of 21 patients with tumors between 5 and 50 mm after MRgFUS for a median period of 14 months and found a single local recurrence.[43] Subsequently, a series in which 24 patients underwent combined treatment with Tamoxifen and HIFU were followed with MR imaging and confirmed with 6-month core biopsy showed a 79% rate of success[40] in the treatment of small tumors. Another study evaluating excised specimens after MRgFUS treatment found that 15 of 28 patients achieved 100% tumor necrosis.[41]

The latter study raises questions about whether less than complete destruction of the tumor would be acceptable for any type of primary therapy. Indeed, incompletely ablated tumor probably equates to positive margins after surgery, which is an indication for mastectomy according to current standards. Despite successful phase II trials in Japan,[43] similar studies in the United States, such as ACRIN, have been stalled, in part for the reasons listed above. Nevertheless, a multicenter trial is currently underway in Europe and Asia aimed at comparing posttreatment MR imaging findings with excision (InSightec).

Regardless of when efficacy and safety trials are conducted, the long-term success of MRgFUS in the treatment of localized breast cancer rests on proof that its efficacy can match conventional therapy. Currently, breast-sparing surgery, lumpectomy, and other surgical procedures have reduced rates of morbidity, maximized successful clinical outcomes, and achieved nearly insurmountable cosmetic results. Once MRgFUS moves beyond the testing stage, the real challenge of recruiting patients into an unproven treatment modality will begin.

Abdominal Organs

Special measures are needed to treat abdominal organs to compensate for respiratory motion. Gating the treatment can be successful if patients are on a ventilator, or potentially, a navigator pulse can be used. In addition, the ribs may limit the approach if the target lesion lies beneath the chest wall.

Liver

Malignancy involving the liver may be either primary or metastatic, but in either case the prognosis is grim, even for localized tumors. In the United States, 40% of patients with hepatocellular carcinoma present with focal lesions but have an expected 5-year survival of 27.7%. Many patients who fail surgical and adjunctive therapies later go on to salvage treatment.

Thermal ablation of primary or metastatic liver tumors, as either adjunctive or salvage therapy, has been well described in treatments such as radiofrequency, microwave, and cryoablation.[44] FUS offers several advantages. Patients with significant restrictions, such as structural liver disease, coagulopathy, or requiring palliation, could safely undergo treatment. It could also potentially be used as a neoadjunctive treatment without altering the surgical approach in smaller lesions.[45,46] Finally, reablation of residual tumor detected on follow-up imaging would not be limited by additional procedural risks or radiation exposure as in other therapies.[47]

The anatomic location of the liver presents significant challenges to successful clinical application of FUS due to several factors: overlying bone obscuring a wide sonographic window, phasic respiratory movement of the liver, and the heat sink effect of the organ's rich vascularity.[48,49] Also, critical nearby anatomy, such as portal structures, bowel, and other upper abdominal organs, are susceptible to far field effects of HIFU, raising a question of how treatment may be safely monitored.[47]

Investigators who pioneered USgFUS have used several approaches to difficult hepatic tumors[50]; however, monitoring with US is beset by limitations discussed in earlier sections. Engineering of MRgFUS systems have been developed to overcome respiratory motion and obstruction by ribs. Newer machines integrate respiratory gating with feedback from transducer elements so that treatment-intensity US energy is transmitted only when a sonographic window is present.[51–54] For such a system to maintain a sufficiently high therapeutic intensity, the number of transducer elements must be sufficiently high to compensate for the number of elements that are switched off as the sonographic window passes along the ribs and intercostal spaces.[47,55]

HIFU for liver tumors to date has been evaluated in the clinical setting primarily using US guidance[50,56]; however, the results are promising. For example, in 1 study USgFUS combined with transcatheter arterial chemoembolization increased survival in the combination group better than transcatheter arterial chemoembolization alone.[56] There have not been significant numbers of patients tested with MRgFUS, although cases have been published.[52]

Major obstacles stand in the way of full clinical evaluation of HIFU for liver tumors. MRgFUS provides the best hope of therapeutic monitoring; however, these techniques remain investigatory and clinical trials are therefore in the future.

Renal

Renal cell carcinoma is a relatively rare disease, with a lifetime incidence of nearly 2%. Sixty-two percent of patients with renal cell carcinoma present at an early, localized stage, attributable to a wider use of cross-sectional imaging over the past 20 years, either by workup for clinical symptoms or as an incidental finding on imaging performed for another purpose.[46,57] The indolent nature of small, noninvasive tumors has led surgeons to alter conventional therapy: where once radical nephrectomy was performed, nephron-sparing surgery is now used. Indeed, focal ablation is used in almost 7% of stage I lesions.[57] A noninvasive alternative renal cell carcinoma treatment would significantly decrease rates of morbidity, for instance, in patients with compromised renal function, in patients with hereditary syndromes, or in elderly persons.[58]

The technical challenges of using HIFU to treat renal tumors are similar to those in the liver because of its proximity to bowel, ribs, the diaphragm, and lung, as well as being subject to respiratory motion.[46] In additional, upper abdominal organs in the far field may also be susceptible to unintended injury. Guidance of HIFU is also complicated by the absorption of the beam by the investing fat of the retroperitoneum, which may present an additional obstacle to targeting lesions successfully on the order of 1 cm, especially in larger patients.[59,60] In fact, to obviate technical challenges, investigators have evaluated laparoscopic FUS, which has shown some success but removes the main advantage of the technique.[60,61] Although monitoring with MR imaging allows the possibility of real-time thermal monitoring, such technology remains investigational and has not been described in the literature.

Safety and feasibility have been demonstrated in USgFUS of renal cell carcinoma in a western population.[60,62] Studies evaluating the treated zone in subsequently excised histopathologic specimens have shown some effectiveness in producing tumor necrosis, but in some samples these changes were absent.[59] Also, in a small clinical trial, 10 of 15 patients with an average tumor size of 2.5 cm were followed for 3 years and were treated successfully.[60] Results of these investigations leave open the possibility that more robust monitoring and guidance such as with MR imaging may produce more promising findings.

Brain

Because of the intricate functional network of the brain, and the often dire prognosis of intracranial tumors or other intracranial lesions, the potential morbidity of neurosurgical intervention weighs heavily in treatment planning. Advances in ablative therapy in the brain have lagged behind treatments elsewhere in the body because of the inherent challenges in dealing not only with the organ itself but also with its surrounding bony skull. FUS may someday allow noninvasive neurosurgical therapy without causing surgical morbidity or the use of ionizing radiation. Applications of FUS in the treatment of brain tumors, ablation for movement disorders, or epilepsy as well as in the delivery of chemotherapy have been investigated.

The main technical challenge of FUS therapy in the brain concerns the skull and its effect on the US beam, which is reflected, absorbed, and distorted by bone. Any successful FUS system must therefore solve the problems of skull penetration by the beam, beam focusing on its target to safely achieve heating, and minimization of the effects of reflected energy on nontarget sites such as the scalp and skull.[63,64] Subsequently, a method for incorporating beam incidence with the variability of the skull shape, density, and thickness was developed using images from a volumetric, thin-slice computed tomographic scan registered to an MR image to eliminate beam defocusing.[63] Using advances in beam steering, an MR-compatible phased array apparatus using more than 500 elements in a hemispheric configuration was developed to fit over the skull, producing a focal spot size of approximately 2 to 4 mm.[64,65]

Three-Tesla MR imaging is used for localization of the lesion to be treated and permits monitoring with thermometry, such as with the system designed by InSightec. Skull and scalp heating is controlled by cycling cooled, degassed water through the transducer, which is fitted tightly over the patient's head.[66] Thermocoagulation in the brain is then achieved during sonication at a threshold temperature of 50°C; however, 100% necrosis is seen between 55°C and 57°C.[67]

The potential for successful noninvasive ablation of a brain neoplasm is perhaps the most compelling application of transcranial MR guided focused ultrasound (tcMRgFUS). Initial feasibility studies successfully induced thermocoagulation in 3 patients with recurrent glioblastome multiforme via a window created by craniotomy, with some clinical success, but also led to a major complication in which 1 patient developed symptoms related to nontarget ablation.[68] Three other patients with glioblastome multiforme were treated without craniotomy in a later trial using the ExAblate 3000 hemispheric transducer developed by InSightec.[69] Significant brain heating was produced in these patients, up to 51°C, and although coagulative necrosis was not achieved in any patient, extrapolation of the data implied that temperatures of at least 55°C could be safely achieved. Unfortunately the next patient in the study suffered a complication and died, and the trial was stopped.[66] It is thought that more focal lesions such as metastases or localized low-grade tumors will be more amenable to tcMRfUS, as glioblastoma has poorly defined borders and infiltrates deeply into surrounding tissues.[66] The future of brain tumor treatment with FUS depends on the ability of prototype machines to continue to incorporate data from continuing studies into subsequent machines to optimize tumor heating within safe limits.

Ablation of smaller foci within the brain has proved to be more successful than larger masses thus far, mainly in the treatment of motor and sensory disorders. Phase I studies have been successfully conducted to determine the feasibility and safety of tcMRgFUS for treatment-resistant chronic neuropathic pain[14] in which 12 patients or 57.9% had improved symptoms after 1 year. Phase I and II trials have been conducted or are underway for the treatment of essential tremor and Parkinson disease.[66] Other applications, such as in the treatment of epilepsy, blood-brain barrier disruption, delivery of chemotherapeutic agents, thrombolysis, and enhancement of radiation treatment,[66] are currently in the preclinical or conceptual stages of development (Figs. 10–12).

FUTURE APPLICATIONS

MRgFUS can be used for a wide variety of applications.

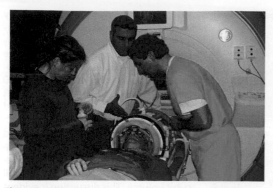

Fig. 10. MRgFUS system with patient seen in the transducer with 1000 element array. The system uses degassed water cooling for the skin and a calculated energy threshold to avoid thermal damage to the skin, bone, and brain cortex. Dr Diane Huss is performing intraoperative testing in the scanner; Eyal Zadicario (engineer from InSightec) and Dr W. Jeff Elias are discussing the transducer alignment during the first FUS treatment of essential tremor, February 25th, 2011. (*Courtesy of* Dr Robert Frysinger, University of Virginia, Charlottesville, VA.)

MRgFUS can be used to lyse clot, which can potentially be used to treat strokes caused by an acute thrombus, and other diseases when clot needs to be lysed.

Drug delivery can be augmented by MRgFUS by creating heat or by mechanical methods. Drugs encapsulated by materials that are either heat sensitive or mechanically sensitive can be locally released at a target where MRFUS either heats the tissue to a desired temperature or mechanically disrupts the carrier. Thermodux is a temperature-sensitive form of Doxirubicin that can be released when the temperature is raised.

Altering tissue permeability that can be used for the brain could potentially be used for gene therapy.

Decreasing the costs by decreasing treatments time and decreasing cost of systems can also aid in this effort.

A major advantage of minimally invasive treatments such as MRgFUS is the decreased pain and recovery time. The recovery time for MRgFUS treatment of fibroid is on the order of hours. Surgical treatments and angiographic uterine artery embolization have recovery times from 1 week to 8 weeks. These treatments are typically covered by health insurance. However, health insurance is not financially responsible for the time patients spend recovering from the procedures and from the time taken off from work. Disability insurance or an employer absorbs the costs of medical leave.

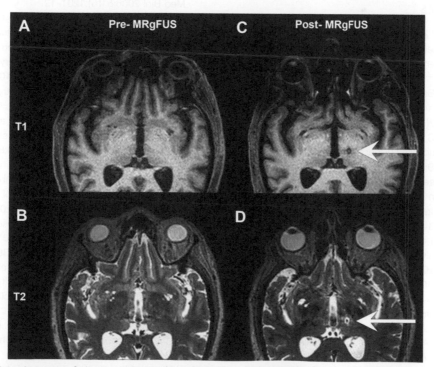

Fig. 11. MR imaging scans from a patient with neuropathic pain. (*A, B*) Pretreatment T1 and T2 axial. (*C, D*) T1 and T2 axials 1 day after MRgFUS treatment with a 2- to 3-mm focal lesion (*arrow*) in the right side of the image in the thalamus. (*Courtesy of* Dr Robert Frysinger, University of Virginia, Charlottesville, VA.)

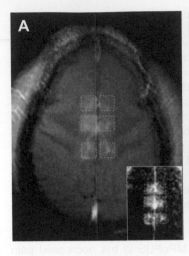
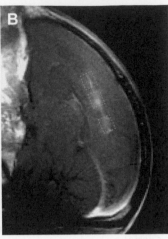

Fig. 12. Blood-brain barrier temporary disruption: contrast-enhanced T1-weighted imaging acquired after sonication of 6 volumes in the cingulate cortex in a rhesus macaque with microbubbles with the ExAblate 4000 (InSightec) clinical transcranial MR imaging-guided focused ultrasound system (*A:* axial; *B:* sagittal). For each volume, the focal point was steered electronically via a phased array transducer to 9 targets in sequence to disrupt the blood-brain barrier in a small cubic volume. This disruption is evident in the images by the delivery of gadolinium diethylenetriamine pentaacetic acid (Magnevist), an MR imaging contrast agent that normally is not delivered to the brain. The acoustic power level used at each volume differed, resulting in different levels of signal enhancement. (*A, inset*) A map of the percentage enhancement in signal intensity relative to imaging acquired before administration of the contrast agent. (*Courtesy of* Nathan McDonald, PhD, and Ferenc Jolesz, MD, PhD, Brigham and Women's Hospital, Boston, MA.)

Widespread adoption of the technology will require sufficient data for applications to support the cost of the treatment and reimbursement from health insurers. Multicenter trials and registries of treated patients will be needed to provide this data.

REFERENCES

1. Lynn JG, Zwemer RL, Chick AJ, et al. A new method for the generation and use of focused ultrasound in experimental biology. J Gen Physiol 1942;26(2): 179–93.

2. Fry WJ, Barnard JW, Fry EJ, et al. Ultrasonic lesions in the mammalian central nervous system. Science 1955;122(3168):179–93.

3. Dogra VS, Zhang M, Bhatt S. High-intensity focused ultrasound (HIFU) therapy applications. Ultrasound Clin 2009;4(3):307–21.

4. Vykhodtseva N, Sorrentino V, Jolesz FA, et al. MRI detection of the thermal effects of focused ultrasound on the brain. Ultrasound Med Biol 2000; 26(5):871–80.

5. Hynynen K, McDannold N, Vykhodtseva N, et al. Noninvasive MR imaging-guided focal opening of the blood-brain barrier in rabbits. Radiology 2001; 220(3):640–6.

6. Jolesz FA, Hynynen K. Magnetic resonance image-guided focused ultrasound surgery. Cancer J 2002;8(Suppl 1):S100–12.

7. Jolesz FA. Future perspectives in intraoperative imaging. Acta Neurochir Suppl 2003;85:7–13.

8. Pennes HH. Analysis of tissue and arterial blood temperatures in the resting human forearm. J Appl Physiol 1948;1(2):93–122.

9. O'Brien WD Jr. Ultrasound-biophysics mechanisms. Prog Biophys Mol Biol 2007;93(1–3):212–55.

10. Hill CR, ter Haar GR. Review article: high intensity focused ultrasound–potential for cancer treatment. Br J Radiol 1995;68(816):1296–303.

11. Arora D, Minor MA, Skliar M, et al. Control of thermal therapies with moving power deposition field. Phys Med Biol 2006;51(5):1201–19.

12. Mougenot C, Salomir R, Palussiere J, et al. Automatic spatial and temporal temperature control for MR-guided focused ultrasound using fast 3D MR thermometry and multispiral trajectory of the focal point. Magn Reson Med 2004;52(5):1005–15.

13. Rieke V, Butts Pauly K. MR thermometry. J Magn Reson Imaging 2008;27(2):376–90.

14. Martin E, Jeanmonod D, Morel A, et al. High-intensity focused ultrasound for noninvasive functional neurosurgery. Ann Neurol 2009;66(6):858–61.

15. Management of Uterine Fibroids. Summary, Evidence Report/Technology Assessment: Number 34. AHRQ Publication No. 01- E051. Rockville (MD): Agency for Healthcare Research and Quality; 2001. Available at: www.ahrq.gov/clinic/epcsums/utersumm.htm.

16. Stewart EA, Shuster LT, Rocca WA. Reassessing hysterectomy. Minn Med 2012;95(3):36–9.

17. Spies JB, Myers ER, Worthington-Kirsch R, et al. The FIBROID Registry: symptom and quality-of-life status 1 year after therapy. Obstet Gynecol 2005;106(6): 1309–18.

18. Wilcox LS, Koonin LM, Pokras R, et al. Hysterectomy in the United States, 1988-1990. Obstet Gynecol 1994;83(4):549–55.

19. Whiteman MK, Hillis SD, Jamieson DJ, et al. Inpatient hysterectomy surveillance in the United States, 2000-2004. Am J Obstet Gynecol 2008;198(1):34.e1–7.

20. Hesley GK, Gorny KR, Woodrum DA. MR-guided focused ultrasound for the treatment of uterine fibroids. Cardiovasc Intervent Radiol 2012. [Epub ahead of print].

21. Gorny KR, Woodrum DA, Brown DL, et al. Magnetic resonance-guided focused ultrasound of uterine leiomyomas: review of a 12-month outcome of 130 clinical patients. J Vasc Interv Radiol 2011;22(6): 857–64.

22. Rabinovici J, David M, Fukunishi H, et al. Pregnancy outcome after magnetic resonance-guided focused ultrasound surgery (MRgFUS) for conservative treatment of uterine fibroids. Fertil Steril 2010; 93(1):199–209.

23. Fukunishi H, Funaki K, Sawada K, et al. Early results of magnetic resonance-guided focused ultrasound surgery of adenomyosis: analysis of 20 cases. J Minim Invasive Gynecol 2008;15(5):571–9.

24. Dong X, Yang Z. High-intensity focused ultrasound ablation of uterine localized adenomyosis. Curr Opin Obstet Gynecol 2010;22(4):326–30.

25. Holmberg L, Bill-Axelson A, Helgesen F, et al. A randomized trial comparing radical prostatectomy with watchful waiting in early prostate cancer. N Engl J Med 2002;347(11):781–9.

26. Djulbegovic M, Beyth RJ, Neuberger MM, et al. Screening for prostate cancer: systematic review and meta-analysis of randomised controlled trials. BMJ 2010;341:c4543.

27. McVey GP, McPhail S, Fowler S, et al. Initial management of low-risk localized prostate cancer in the UK: analysis of the British Association of Urological Surgeons Cancer Registry. BJU Int 2010;106(8): 1161–4.

28. Cooperberg MR, Broering JM, Carroll PR. Time trends and local variation in primary treatment of localized prostate cancer. J Clin Oncol 2010;28(7): 1117–23.

29. Tempany C, Straus S, Hata N, et al. MR-guided prostate interventions. J Magn Reson Imaging 2008; 27(2):356–67.

30. Chopra R, Burtnyk M, N'Djin WA, et al. MRI-controlled transurethral ultrasound therapy for localised prostate cancer. Int J Hyperthermia 2010;26(8): 804–21.

31. Rouviere O, Glas L, Girouin N, et al. Prostate cancer ablation with transrectal high-intensity focused ultrasound: assessment of tissue destruction with contrast-enhanced US. Radiology 2011;259(2): 583–91.

32. Tempany CM, McDannold NJ, Hynynen K, et al. Focused ultrasound surgery in oncology: overview and principles. Radiology 2011;259(1):39–56.

33. Warmuth M, Johansson T, Mad P. Systematic review of the efficacy and safety of high-intensity focussed ultrasound for the primary and salvage treatment of prostate cancer. Eur Urol 2010;58(6):803–15.

34. Heidenreich A, Bellmunt J, Bolla M, et al. EAU guidelines on prostate cancer. Part 1: screening, diagnosis, and treatment of clinically localised disease. Eur Urol 2011;59(1):61–71.

35. Liberman B, Gianfelice D, Inbar Y, et al. Pain palliation in patients with bone metastases using MR-guided focused ultrasound surgery: a multicenter study. Ann Surg Oncol 2009;16(1):140–6.

36. Chen W, Zhu H, Zhang L, et al. Primary bone malignancy: effective treatment with high-intensity focused ultrasound ablation. Radiology 2010; 255(3):967–78.

37. Siegel R, Naishadham D, Jemal A. Cancer statistics, 2012. CA Cancer J Clin 2012;62(1):10–29.

38. Darby S, McGale P, Correa C, et al. Effect of radiotherapy after breast-conserving surgery on 10-year recurrence and 15-year breast cancer death: meta-analysis of individual patient data for 10,801 women in 17 randomised trials. Lancet 2011; 378(9804):1707–16.

39. Litiere S, Werutsky G, Fentiman IS, et al. Breast conserving therapy versus mastectomy for stage I-II breast cancer: 20 year follow-up of the EORTC 10801 phase 3 randomised trial. Lancet Oncol 2012;13(4):412–9.

40. Gianfelice D, Khiat A, Amara M, et al. MR imaging-guided focused US ablation of breast cancer: histopathologic assessment of effectiveness–initial experience. Radiology 2003;227(3):849–55.

41. Furusawa H, Namba K, Thomsen S, et al. Magnetic resonance-guided focused ultrasound surgery of breast cancer: reliability and effectiveness. J Am Coll Surg 2006;203(1):54–63.

42. Brenin DR. Focused ultrasound ablation for the treatment of breast cancer. Ann Surg Oncol 2011;18(11): 3088–94.

43. Furusawa H, Namba K, Nakahara H, et al. The evolving non-surgical ablation of breast cancer: MR guided focused ultrasound (MRgFUS). Breast Cancer 2007;14(1):55–8.

44. Lau WY, Ho SK, Yu SC, et al. Salvage surgery following downstaging of unresectable hepatocellular carcinoma. Ann Surg 2004;240(2):299–305.

45. Jolesz FA, Hynynen K, McDannold N, et al. Noninvasive thermal ablation of hepatocellular carcinoma by using magnetic resonance imaging-guided focused ultrasound. Gastroenterology 2004;127(5 Suppl 1): S242–7.

46. Gedroyc WM. New clinical applications of magnetic resonance-guided focused ultrasound. Top Magn Reson Imaging 2006;17(3):189–94.

47. Jolesz FA. MRI-guided focused ultrasound surgery. Annu Rev Med 2009;60:417–30.

48. Ng KK, Poon RT, Chan SC, et al. High-intensity focused ultrasound for hepatocellular carcinoma: a single-center experience. Ann Surg 2011;253(5): 981–7.

49. Wu F, Wang ZB, Chen WZ, et al. Extracorporeal high intensity focused ultrasound ablation in the treatment of 1038 patients with solid carcinomas in China: an overview. Ultrason Sonochem 2004;11(3-4):149–54.

50. Orsi F, Zhang L, Arnone P, et al. High-intensity focused ultrasound ablation: effective and safe therapy for solid tumors in difficult locations. AJR Am J Roentgenol 2010;195(3):W245–52.

51. Braunewell S, Gunther M, Preusser T. Toward focused ultrasound liver surgery under free breathing. Crit Rev Biomed Eng 2012;40(3):221–34.

52. Okada A, Murakami T, Mikami K, et al. A case of hepatocellular carcinoma treated by MR-guided focused ultrasound ablation with respiratory gating. Magn Reson Med Sci 2006;5(3):167–71.

53. Tokuda J, Morikawa S, Haque HA, et al. Adaptive 4D MR imaging using navigator-based respiratory signal for MRI-guided therapy. Magn Reson Med 2008;59(5):1051–61.

54. Holbrook AB, Santos JM, Kaye E, et al. Real-time MR thermometry for monitoring HIFU ablations of the liver. Magn Reson Med 2010;63(2):365–73.

55. Daum DR, Smith NB, King R, et al. In vivo demonstration of noninvasive thermal surgery of the liver and kidney using an ultrasonic phased array. Ultrasound Med Biol 1999;25(7):1087–98.

56. Wu F, Wang ZB, Chen WZ, et al. Advanced hepatocellular carcinoma: treatment with high-intensity focused ultrasound ablation combined with transcatheter arterial embolization. Radiology 2005; 235(2):659–67.

57. Cooperberg MR, Mallin K, Kane CJ, et al. Treatment trends for stage I renal cell carcinoma. J Urol 2011; 186(2):394–9.

58. Olweny EO, Cadeddu JA. Novel methods for renal tissue ablation. Curr Opin Urol 2012;22:379–84.

59. Nabi G, Goodman C, Melzer A. High intensity focused ultrasound treatment of small renal masses: Clinical effectiveness and technological advances. Indian J Urol 2010;26(3):331–7.

60. Ritchie RW, Leslie T, Phillips R, et al. Extracorporeal high intensity focused ultrasound for renal tumours: a 3-year follow-up. BJU Int 2010;106(7):1004–9.

61. Klingler HC, Susani M, Seip R, et al. A novel approach to energy ablative therapy of small renal tumours: laparoscopic high-intensity focused ultrasound. Eur Urol 2008;53(4):810–6 [discussion: 817–8].

62. Illing RO, Kennedy JE, Wu F, et al. The safety and feasibility of extracorporeal high-intensity focused ultrasound (HIFU) for the treatment of liver and kidney tumours in a Western population. Br J Cancer 2005;93(8):890–5.

63. Clement GT, Sun J, Hynynen K. The role of internal reflection in transskull phase distortion. Ultrasonics 2001;39(2):109–13.

64. Clement GT. Modeling of transcranial ultrasound for therapeutic and diagnostic applications. J Acoust Soc Am 2012;132(3):1927.

65. Clement GT, White PJ, King RL, et al. A magnetic resonance imaging-compatible, large-scale array for trans-skull ultrasound surgery and therapy. J Ultrasound Med 2005;24(8):1117–25.

66. Medel R, Monteith SJ, Elias WJ, et al. Magnetic resonance-guided focused ultrasound surgery: part 2: a review of current and future applications. Neurosurgery 2012;71(4):755–63.

67. Jeanmonod D, Werner B, Morel A, et al. Transcranial magnetic resonance imaging-guided focused ultrasound: noninvasive central lateral thalamotomy for chronic neuropathic pain. Neurosurg Focus 2012; 32(1):E1.

68. Ram Z, Cohen ZR, Harnof S, et al. Magnetic resonance imaging-guided, high-intensity focused ultrasound for brain tumor therapy. Neurosurgery 2006; 59(5):949–55 [discussion: 955–6].

69. McDannold N, Clement GT, Black P, et al. Transcranial magnetic resonance imaging- guided focused ultrasound surgery of brain tumors: initial findings in 3 patients. Neurosurgery 2010;66(2):323–32 [discussion: 332].

Duplex Ultrasonography in the Management of Varicose Veins

Ashwani K. Sharma, MD*, Douglas Drumsta, MD,
David E. Lee, MD

KEYWORDS

- Duplex ultrasonography • Reflux • Ultrasound-guided ablation • Ultrasound-guided sclerotherapy

KEY POINTS

- Most patients with varicose veins do not undergo a proper workup before treatment.
- Advancements in duplex ultrasonography have helped to better understand the pathophysiology of varicose veins.
- With ultrasound guidance, most of the varicose vein procedures can now be done on an outpatient basis safely and efficiently.

 Videos of thermal ablation of varicose veins accompany this article

BACKGROUND

Varicose veins are a common condition that affects both men and women. Some studies suggest prevalence rates of up to 56% in men and up to 73% in women.[1] Varicose veins are thought to be primarily a cosmetic condition; however, as the disease progresses, it could become symptomatic and can lead to venous ulcerations (**Fig. 1**).[2,3] Treatment costs are estimated at approximately $3 billion a year, and a total of 2 million work-days are lost yearly.[2] Multiple diagnostic modalities such as phlebography, conventional venography, light reflux rheography, and air plethysmography among others are used in the diagnosis of varicose veins. Duplex ultrasonography has emerged as the preferred imaging modality in the management of patients with varicose veins.[4]

ANATOMY

Veins of the lower extremity are divided into 3 categories: superficial, perforating, and deep veins. Normally, flow should be in the cephalad direction and drain from the superficial to the deep venous system. The deep veins are located deep to the muscle fascia in the legs and drain blood from muscles and blood that they receive from the superficial venous system via the perforating veins.[5] Reflux in the greater saphenous vein (GSV) is found in about 75% to 80% of limbs with chronic venous disease (**Fig. 2**A) and that in small saphenous vein (SSV) (see **Fig. 2**B) and nonsaphenous veins is found in 10% (see **Fig. 2**C); however, the latter value can reach 20% in patients presenting with recurrent varicose veins.[6]

GSV is the largest of the superficial veins. This vein begins as the continuation of the dorsal venous arch in the foot, travels anterior to the medial malleolus, and ascends the medial aspect of the leg, ultimately draining into the deep system at the saphenofemoral junction (SFJ). The GSV can be partially duplicated in approximately 20% of cases.[5] The GSV is easily identified particularly in the proximal to middle thigh region because of

Statement of funding support and financial disclosure: There is no financial support provided for this project. The above-mentioned authors have no financial disclosure to report.
Department of Imaging Sciences, University of Rochester, 601 Elmwood Avenue, Rochester, NY 14642, USA
* Corresponding author.
E-mail address: Ashwani_Sharma@urmc.rochester.edu

Ultrasound Clin 8 (2013) 227–235
http://dx.doi.org/10.1016/j.cult.2012.12.008
1556-858X/13/$ – see front matter © 2013 Elsevier Inc. All rights reserved.

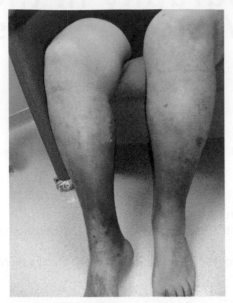

Fig. 1. Patient with bilateral lower-extremity varicose veins presented with skin changes after venous hypertension.

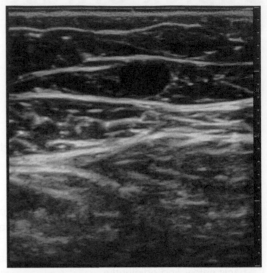

Fig. 3. "Saphenous eye" appearance of the greater saphenous vein in the axial section of ultrasonographic image.

its typical ultrasonographic appearance known as the saphenous eye (**Fig. 3**).[7] A total of 5 anatomic GSV variations have been reported depending on whether it is single or duplicated (**Fig. 4**) and the presence/duplication of its tributaries.[8]

The SSV begins on the lateral aspect of the foot, travels posterior to the lateral malleolus, and ascends the midline of the calf superficial to the muscular fascia and deep to the saphenous fascia. In approximately two-thirds of patients, the SSV drains entirely into the popliteal vein just above the knee via the saphenopopliteal junction (SPJ). In as many as one-third of the patients, the SSV drains into a posterior medial tributary of the GSV, directly into the GSV (as the vein of Giacomini) (**Fig. 5**), or into a deep vein in the thigh via a perforator.[5] Over the years, there have been different classifications of the SPJ, the first being, low and high terminations. A newer simpler classification describes just 3 groups. Group A comprises the classical SPJ, group B comprises

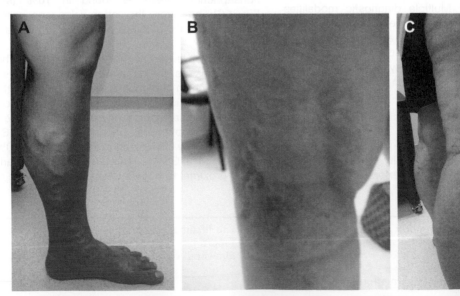

Fig. 2. Typical distribution of greater saphenous (*A*), lesser saphenous (*B*), and nonsaphenous (*C*) varicose veins.

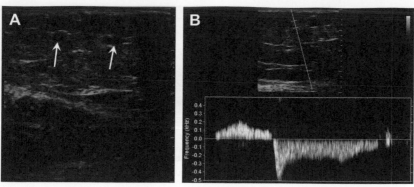

Fig. 4. Duplicated GSV (*arrows*) on gray scale ultrasonography (*A*) with reflux on spectral Doppler (*B*).

those with a "connection to the deep stem more cranially," and group C contains all cases with an existing upward extension of the SSV without connection to the popliteal deep venous system.[9] By definition, the perforator veins pierce deep fascia and connect superficial veins to the muscular and the deep venous systems (**Fig. 6**).

PATHOPHYSIOLOGY

The cause of varicose veins is multifactorial and may include increased intravenous pressure caused by prolonged standing, increased intraabdominal pressure, familial and congenital factors,

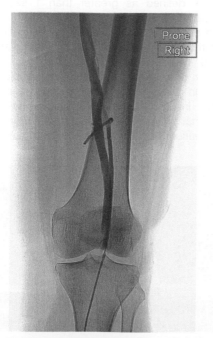

Fig. 5. Conventional venography showing SSV draining directly into the GSV.

deep venous thrombosis, or less commonly, arteriovenous shunting.[10,11]

The earliest theory regarding the pathophysiology of varicose veins was based on venous valvular incompetence. The incompetent valves result in venous hypertension in the more caudal segments, resulting in the classical clinical picture.[12] The primary venous wall weakness theory hypothesizes that abnormalities in the venous wall lead to the development of varicose veins. Microscopic analysis of varicose veins uniformly reveals intimal hypertrophy, luminal dilatation, wall thickening, and disruption of the normal extracellular matrix and smooth muscle cells.[2] Tissue cultures from varicosities have demonstrated an overproduction of type I collagen and an underproduction of type III collagen in the extracellular matrix. Furthermore, there is a decrease in the elastin/collagen ratio and a decreased number of smooth muscle cells.[2,12] Although the pathophysiology of varicose veins is not completely understood, it likely involves a combination of factors including mechanical abnormalities, such as incompetent valves and venous hypertension, alterations of the venous wall composition at the microscopic level.

DIAGNOSIS

Duplex ultrasonography has become the primary imaging modality for the evaluation of varicose veins (**Box 1**). The role of ultrasonography is to identify the source and course of varicosities and to assess the veins preprocedurally. The sensitivity and positive predictive value for the clinical diagnosis of venous insufficiency in varicose veins is only 32% and 24%, respectively.[13] It is imperative to evaluate the entire venous system because some patients may have superficial venous insufficiency due to primary deep venous incompetence or reflux or secondary superficial insufficiency

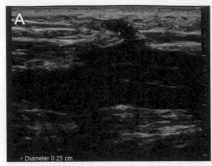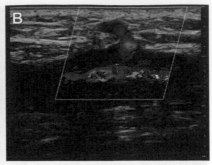

Fig. 6. Gray scale (*A*) and color flow (*B*) ultrasonography showing a dilated tortuous perforator with reflux.

due to postthrombotic states, which can affect the long-term treatment outcome.[11] Evaluation of superficial veins should be performed in the standing position with the extremity that is being examined in a non–weight-bearing position because such positioning increases the sensitivity and specificity.

The examination is performed with multifrequency linear array high-frequency ultrasound transducer (4–7 MHz).[14] The recommended preoperative evaluation as per the Union Internationale de Phlébologie (UIP) includes evaluation of the deep venous system, including the popliteal and common femoral vein, for patency and reflux. The perforating veins and main superficial trunks, including the GSV, lesser saphenous vein, anterior accessory saphenous vein, posterior accessory saphenous vein, and Giacomini vein, should be evaluated for their diameter and assessed for reflux. In addition, tributaries and nonsaphenous veins should be evaluated for competency and the SFJ and SPJ should be evaluated for reflux.[11] Distinct areas of reflux can be found in veins that are not part of the GSV or SSV in 10% of patients.[15] Valsalva and compression maneuvers are used when reflux is not obvious (**Fig. 7**). GSV and SSV are traced down to define the course of the vein, its tributaries, the perforators, and the extent of reflux. Anatomic variations are very

common in the venous system and need to be documented. Sometimes, conventional venography is done to confirm duplex ultrasonographic findings.

The upper limits of normal for the diameter of the GSV and the lesser saphenous vein in the upright position are 4 mm and 3 mm, respectively. Varicosities exhibit dilatation beyond these measurements, sometimes upward of 15 mm (**Fig. 8**).[5] Reflux, rather than size, is a better indicator of the disease.

Normal competent venous valves allow for a small amount of reflux (**Fig. 9**). To distinguish competent from incompetent valves, more than 0.5 seconds of reversal of flow is used to define venous reflux in the superficial venous system, deep femoral vein, and deep calf veins. Venous reflux in the common femoral, femoral, and popliteal veins is defined as greater than 1 second of reversal of flow (see **Fig. 7**). Reflux in the perforating system is defined as reversal of flow for more than 0.35 seconds.[16] Other parameters that should be obtained include the peak reflux velocity, peak reflux flow, and venous diameter. Although reflux duration is a good marker for venous insufficiency, several studies have indicated that the peak reflux velocity is a more accurate measurement of the severity of disease.[11]

Box 1
Preprocedure duplex imaging both when standing and when lying down

Deep venous assessment for thrombosis and reflux

Terminal valve reflux of SFJ and SPJ

Diameter and extent of reflux in GSV and SSV

Diameter and reflux in perforating veins

Diameter and reflux in nonsaphenous veins

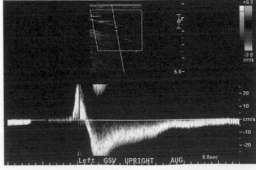

Fig. 7. Spectral Doppler showing prolonged reflux in GSV on compression maneuver. AUG, augmentation.

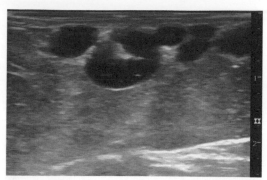

Fig. 8. Dilated tortuous varicose veins on ultrasonography.

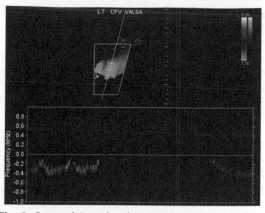

Fig. 9. Spectral Doppler showing no evidence of reflux even after Valsalva maneuver. LT, left; CFV, common femoral vein.

TREATMENT MODALITIES
Sclerotherapy

The principle of sclerotherapy is that a sclerosing agent causes endothelial damage by multiple mechanisms associated with a decrease in endothelial cell surface tension, interference with cell surface lipids, disruption of intercellular cements, and extraction of the cell surface proteins.[17] Ultimately, the endothelial and vessel wall damage results in obliteration of the vein into a thread of connective tissue. Foam sclerosants concentrate their effects on the intima more intensely than liquid sclerosants, and thus are more promising than liquid sclerosants in the treatment of venous insufficiency.[18] Ultrasound-guided sclerotherapy can be easily and effectively performed in an outpatient clinical setting with minimal adverse effects (**Fig. 10**).[19]

Ultrasonography is used to direct sclerosants into deeper superficial veins and incompetent perforating veins that cannot be accurately identified by the naked eye. Identification of incompetent vein segments and distinction of these from adjoining normal structures improves the success and minimizes the risk of extravasation. The target vein is first punctured with real-time ultrasound guidance and then monitored during injection of the sclerosant by visualizing microbubbles of the sclerosant, which produces echoes. This effect is much more pronounced when foam sclerosants are used (see **Fig. 10**). In addition, ultrasonography is used to observe vasospasm, which has a correlation with a positive therapeutic outcome.[20]

Thermal Ablation

Thermal ablation has largely replaced surgical high ligation with or without stripping for saphenous

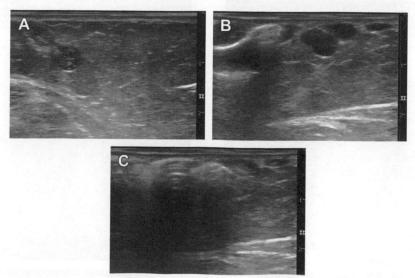

Fig. 10. (A–C). Ultrasonographic image showing controlled progressive increase in echogenic shadows in the varicose vein during foam sclerosant injection. Injection should be stopped if there is evidence of extravasation.

veins in the United States. Endovascular laser therapy (EVLT) and radiofrequency ablation (RFA) have been used for the treatment of saphenous vein incompetence. RFA delivers radiofrequency energy to achieve heat-induced venous spasm and collagen shrinkage, whereas EVLT releases thermal energy both to the blood and to the venous wall, causing localized tissue damage.[21]

Ultrasonography plays a pivotal role in thermal ablation. The lowest incompetent venous segment is accessed under ultrasound guidance followed by placement of sheath and subsequently, the probe. Positioning of the probe, at or below a competent superficial epigastric vein or 10 to 20 mm distal to the SFJ, is done using ultrasound guidance (**Fig. 11**, Video 1). The catheter can be made more echogenic by inserting a J wire into it, which helps in better visualization with ultrasonography.

Perivenous tumescent anesthesia, which is a very important part of the procedure, must be done under ultrasound guidance (**Fig. 12** and Video 2). This anesthesia works by making the procedure painless, preventing vasospasm, and ensuring venous compression for good results. The authors always macerate the segment of vein proximal to the sheath under ultrasound guidance by multiple punctures with a needle (Video 3). The authors believe that it causes spasm of the

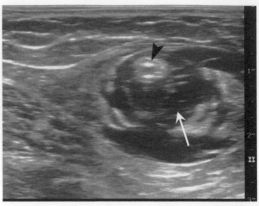

Fig. 12. Transaxial ultrasonographic image demonstrating a halo of tumescent fluid (*arrow*) surrounding the GSV (*arrowhead*).

vein and helps in preventing the propagation of the thrombus into the femoral veins.

Delivery of thermal energy begins after ultrasonography is used to confirm that the tip of the ablative tool is at the desired starting point (**Fig. 13**). With the laser devices, steam bubble generation can be identified with ultrasonography after the procedure (**Fig. 14**, Video 4).

Phlebectomy

The ambulatory phlebectomy procedure eliminates varicose veins through a series of small punctures made in the skin adjacent to the vein. The varicose vein is then removed in small segments. The veins are detected mainly visually

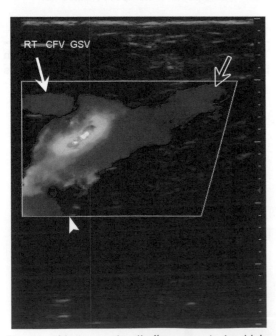

Fig. 11. Ablation probe (*hollow arrow*) should be placed distal to the superficial epigastric vein (*arrow*) and not just to the saphenofemoral junction (*arrowhead*).

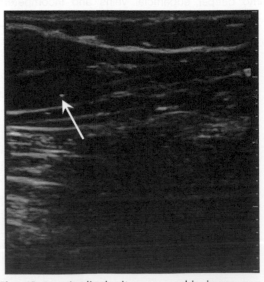

Fig. 13. Longitudinal ultrasonographic image confirming the echogenic tip (*arrow*) of the laser probe at the right location before starting the ablation.

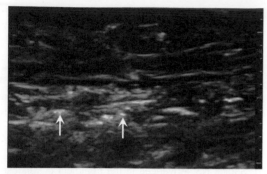

Fig. 14. Steam bubbles (*arrows*) noted in the ablated vein after the procedure on ultrasonography.

for the procedure. However, vein light and duplex ultrasonography are also useful when the vein can be difficult to see when collapsed in supine/prone position.

POSTPROCEDURAL FOLLOW-UP

The purpose of follow-up duplex ultrasonography after treatment is to assess for adequacy of the initial treatment, to detect any complication early, and to identify the possible need for any further treatment by defining the new baseline (**Box 2**).

The UIP consensus document[14] recommends immediate ultrasonography after 1 to 4 weeks of surgery or thermal ablation to check if the intended immediate goal has been achieved. Ultrasonography also helps in defining a new baseline for future and also detecting posttreatment deep venous thrombosis. The UIP also recommends immediate ultrasonography after treatment as part of sequential treatments, such as staged foam sclerotherapy and combined procedures.

Studies have shown that the frequency of deep venous thrombosis posttreatment varies with the study protocol; when ultrasonography was

> **Box 2**
> **Posttreatment duplex ultrasonographic imaging protocol**
>
> Immediate: 1 to 4 weeks after procedure
> Late:
>> Short term (1 year)
>> Midterm (2–3 years)
>> Long term (5 years)

performed only in symptomatic patients, the incidence was 0.1% to 0.2%, but when it was done systematically, the incidence increased to 1.1% to 1.8%.[22,23] Some people think that even a small thrombus in the deep venous system is pathologic,[24] but the authors usually follow-up non–flow-limiting small thrombus extending into the deep venous system with ultrasonography. The authors have seen these acute thrombi shrink back into the superficial veins (**Fig. 15**).

The UIP recommends[14] late ultrasonographic follow-up at 1 year (short-term, for predicting long-term outcome), 2 to 3 years (mid-term), and 5 years (long-term, for development of recurrence).

Early examination of the treated vein demonstrates a smaller diameter, no flow, and hyperechoic wall thickening.[25] The wall thickening (**Fig. 16**) usually obliterates the lumen, has low-level echoes, and is incompressible.[26] These findings can be distinguished from a thrombus, which appears as a hypoechoic to moderately hyperechoic filling defect in a vein that is dilated, rather than shrunken, compared with its preprocedural appearance. Imaging performed approximately 3–6 months after the procedure shows that the treated veins are significantly diminished in size and may be difficult to identify.[25] Treatment failure is usually identified in the first few months as either

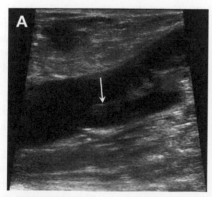
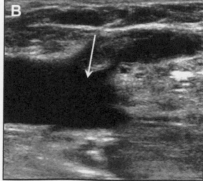

Fig. 15. (*A*) One-week postablation longitudinal ultrasonographic image showing extension of thrombus beyond the saphenofemoral junction (*arrow*). (*B*) One-month follow-up ultrasonographic image shows thrombus retracting back into the GSV (*arrow*).

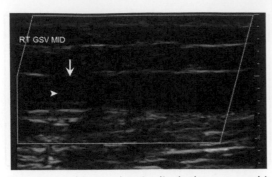

Fig. 16. Postablation, longitudinal ultrasonographic image of GSV shows thickening of GSV wall (*arrow*) with no flow because of thrombus (*arrowhead*).

thrombosed venous segments that recanalize or as those that appear unchanged from the pretreatment appearance.[25]

SUMMARY

Duplex ultrasonography helps in greater understanding of the anatomy and pathophysiology of superficial varicose veins. Duplex ultrasonography has become an integral part in the management of patients with varicose veins. Correct anatomic variation, course of the veins with the extent of reflux, and flow mapping is required before planning treatment in all patients with varicose veins. Treatment with thermal ablation, sclerotherapy, and occasionally phlebectomy require monitoring with duplex ultrasonography. Once treated, all patients are followed up using immediate and late ultrasonography.

VIDEOS

Videos related to this article can be found online at http://dx.doi.org/10.1016/j.cult.2012.12.008.

REFERENCES

1. Beebe-Dimmer JL, Pfeifer JR, Engle JS, et al. The epidemiology of chronic venous insufficiency and varicose veins. Ann Epidemiol 2005;15(3):175–84.
2. Oklu R, Habito R, Mayr M, et al. Pathogenesis of varicose veins. J Vasc Interv Radiol 2012;23(1): 33–9.
3. Khilnani N. Clinical evaluation of the patients with lower extremity venous insufficiency. J Vasc Interv Radiol 2005;16(Suppl 2):P241–3.
4. Ruckley CV, Evans CJ, Allan PL, et al. Chronic venous insufficiency: clinical and duplex correlations. The Edinburgh Vein Study of venous disorders in the general population. J Vasc Surg 2002;36(3):520–5.
5. Min RJ, Khilnani NM, Golia P. Duplex ultrasound evaluation of lower extremity venous insufficiency. J Vasc Interv Radiol 2003;14(10):1233–41.
6. Perrin MR, Labropoulos N, Leon LR Jr. Presentation of the patient with recurrent varices after surgery (REVAS). J Vasc Surg 2006;43(2):327–34 [discussion: 334].
7. Bailly M. Cartographie CHIVA. Paris: Enclyclopedie Medico-Chirurgicale; 1993. p. 43–161-B: 1–4.
8. Ricci S, Caggiati A. Echoanatomical patterns of the long saphenous vein in patients with primary varices and in healthy subjects. Phlebology 1999;14:54–8.
9. Caggiati A. Fascial relationships of the short saphenous vein. J Vasc Surg 2001;34:241–6.
10. Sadick NS. Advances in the treatment of varicose veins: ambulatory phlebectomy, foam sclerotherapy, endovascular laser, and radiofrequency closure [review]. Dermatol Clin 2005;23(3):443–55, vi.
11. Jones RH, Carek PJ. Management of varicose veins [review]. Am Fam Physician 2008;78(11):1289–94.
12. Fan C. Venous pathophysiology. Semin Intervent Radiol 2005;22(3):157–61.
13. De Maeseneer M, Pichot O, Cavezzi A, et al. Duplex ultrasound investigation of the veins of the lower limbs after treatment for varicose veins – UIP consensus document. Eur J Vasc Endovasc Surg 2011;42(1):89–102.
14. Gillespie D, Glass C. Importance of ultrasound evaluation in the diagnosis of venous insufficiency: guidelines and techniques. Semin Vasc Surg 2010; 23(2):85–9.
15. Labropoulos N, Tiongson J, Pryor L, et al. Nonsaphenous superficial vein reflux. J Vasc Surg 2001; 34(5):872–7.
16. Labropoulos N, Tiongson J, Pryor L, et al. Definition of venous reflux in lower-extremity veins. J Vasc Surg 2003;38(4):793–8.
17. Duffy DM. Sclerosants: a comparative review [review]. Dermatol Surg 2010;36(Suppl 2):1010–25.
18. Yamaki T, Nozaki M, Iwasaka S. Comparative study of duplex-guided foam sclerotherapy and duplex-guided liquid sclerotherapy for the treatment of superficial venous insufficiency. Dermatol Surg 2004;30(5):718–22 [discussion: 722].
19. Hamahata A, Yamaki T, Sakurai H. Outcomes of ultrasound-guided foam sclerotherapy for varicose veins of the lower extremities: a single center experience. Dermatol Surg 2011;37(6):804–9.
20. Stucker M, Kobus S, Altmeyer P, et al. Review of published information on foam sclerotherapy. Dermatol Surg 2010;36:983–92.
21. Puggioni A, Kalra M, Carmo M, et al. Endovenous laser therapy and radiofrequency ablation of the great saphenous vein: analysis of early efficacy and complications. J Vasc Surg 2005;42(3):488–93.
22. Guex JJ, Allaert FA, Gillet JL, et al. Immediate and midterm complications of sclerotherapy: report of a prospective multicenter registry of 12,173 sclerotherapy sessions. Dermatol Surg 2005;31(2):123–8 [discussion: 128].

23. Guex JJ. Complications and side-effects of foam scle-rotherapy [review]. Phlebology 2009;24(6):270–4.

24. Mozes G, Kalra M, Carmo M, et al. Extension of saphenous thrombus into the femoral vein: a potential complication of new endovenous ablation tech-niques. J Vasc Surg 2005;41(1):130–5.

25. Min RJ. Common clinical patterns and duplex evalu-ation of venous insufficiency. J Vasc Interv Radiol 2005;16(Suppl 2):P144–6.

26. Min RJ, Khilnani N, Zimmet SE. Endovenous laser treatment of saphenous vein reflux: long-term results. J Vasc Interv Radiol 2003;14(8):991–6.

Ultrasound Imaging and Interventional Treatment of Portal Vein Thrombosis

Katherine Kaproth-Joslin, MD, PhD*,
Ashwani K. Sharma, MD, Deborah J. Rubens, MD

KEYWORDS

- Portal vein • Thrombosis • Ultrasound • Interventional radiology • Acute thrombus
- Chronic thrombus

KEY POINTS

- Ultrasound is the preferred imaging modality for the study of acquired abnormalities of the portal venous system, including acute and chronic portal vein thrombosis.
- Recanalization of the portal venous system is not always accomplished by medical management alone.
- Multiple interventional radiology techniques are available in the management of acute and chronic portal venous thrombosis and are often used in combination.

BACKGROUND

Portal vein thrombosis (PVT) is defined as the complete or partial obstruction of the portal vein and occurs secondary to disturbance of Virchow triad, including reduced flow, hypercoagulability, and endothelial disturbance.[1,2] In the United States, cirrhotic liver disease is the most common cause of a reduced portal blood flow with other entities such as hepatobiliary malignancies and gastric carcinoma also producing a decrease in portal velocity. There are many conditions that create a hypercoagulable state, including inherited prothrombotic conditions, malignancy, dehydration, and trauma. Finally, endothelial disturbances in the portal vein often occur secondary to local inflammation and infection, including conditions such as pancreatitis, abdominal surgery, ascending cholangitis.

PVT is typically divided into the two general clinical categories of acute and chronic PVT, but the separation can be somewhat subjective and clinically it may be difficult to distinguish between the two entities.[3] Acute portal vein thrombosis is considered in patients who become symptomatic less than 60 days before medical assessment and who do not have evidence of collateral circulation or portal hypertension.[4] Symptoms are dependent on extent of the obstruction and speed of the thrombus development and individuals with partial or slowly developing thrombus of the portal venous system may be asymptomatic. For symptomatic individuals, commonly described findings include transient abdominal pain, fever, nonspecific dyspeptic symptoms, and diarrhea. High morbidity and mortality can occur if acute portal vein thrombosis is associated with progressive intestinal ischemia, producing severe abdominal

Statement of funding support and financial disclosure: There is no financial support provided for this project. The authors have no financial disclosure to report.
Department of Imaging Sciences, University of Rochester Medical Center, University of Rochester, 601 Elmwood Avenue, Box 648, Rochester, NY 14642, USA
* Corresponding author.
E-mail address: Katherine_kaproth-Joslin@urmc.rochester.edu

Ultrasound Clin 8 (2013) 237–247
http://dx.doi.org/10.1016/j.cult.2012.12.012
1556-858X/13/$ – see front matter © 2013 Elsevier Inc. All rights reserved.

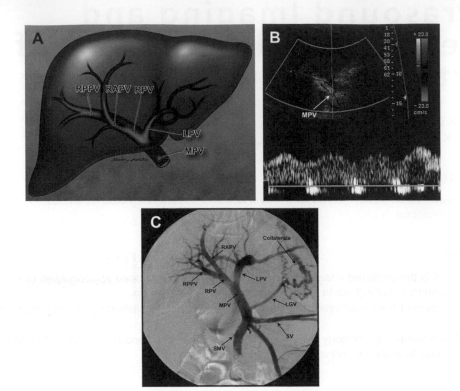

Fig. 1. Normal portal vein anatomy. (*A*) Classic portal vein anatomy. (*B*) Color spectral Doppler ultrasound imaging of the main portal vein. Image demonstrates forward hepatopetal flow into the liver with an average velocity of 23 cm per second. Note the phasicity of the portal vein secondary to respiratory variation. (*C*) Venography of the portal vein in a patient with cirrhosis. Note the gastric collateral vessels. LGV, Left gastric vein; LPV, left portal vein; MPV, main portal vein; RAPV, right anterior portal vein; RPPV, right posterior portal vein; RPV, right portal vein; SMV, superior mesenteric vein; SV, splenic vein.

pain, hematochezia, ascites, metabolic acidosis, peritonitis, renal, and/or respiratory failure.

Progression to chronic portal vein thrombosis occurs when hepatopetal collateral veins begin to develop, allowing blood to bypass the obstructed portion of the portal vein, leading to what is called cavernous transformation of the porta hepatis.[4] This condition often occurs in the

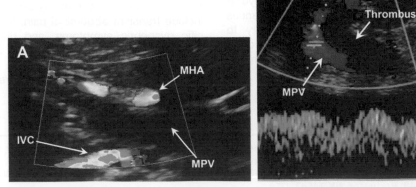

Fig. 2. Acute thrombosis of the portal vein. Color Doppler ultrasound images of the main portal vein. (*A*) Occlusive hypoechoic thrombus of the main portal vein (MPV) with expected color flow in the main hepatic artery (MHA). (*B*) Nonocclusive hypoechoic thrombus of the MPV, with expected portal vein spectral Doppler waveform in the patent portion of the vessel. IVC, Inferior vena cava.

setting of cirrhosis with signs and symptoms primarily related to portal hypertension, including ascites, gastrointestinal bleeding, splenomegaly, and hypersplenism.

IMAGING
Normal Portal Vein Imaging

The hepatic portal vein supplies approximately 75% of the blood flow to the liver, with the remaining 25% of the liver blood supply provided by the hepatic artery. The portal vein is formed from the confluence of the superior mesenteric and splenic veins, with additional drainage from the inferior mesenteric, gastric, and cystic veins. Just before reaching the liver, the main portal vein divides into right and left portal veins, which subsequently divide into smaller branches, ultimately emptying into the hepatic sinusoids (**Fig. 1**A).

Ultrasound is the imaging modality of choice for assessing portal vein thrombosis, evaluating direction, velocity, and phasicity of blood flow. The normal portal vein demonstrates hepatopetal flow into the liver, with minor respiratory phasicity. Spectral Doppler velocities are relatively low, between 15 and 40 cm per second (see **Fig. 1**B).

Venography of the portal vein is typically performed via a transjugular approach. In this method,

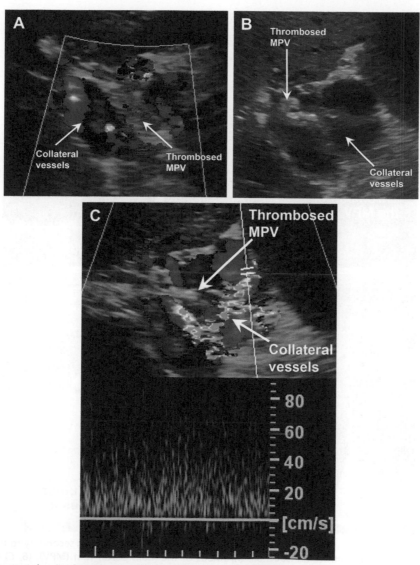

Fig. 3. Chronic portal vein thrombosis with cavernous transformation. Cavernous transformation of the main portal vein. (*A*) Color Doppler and (*B*) grayscale images demonstrate multiple hypoechoic collateral vessels twisting around the echogenic chronic thrombus in the main portal vein (MPV). (*C*) Spectral tracing in a collateral demonstrates a hepatopetal venous waveform.

the jugular vein is accessed and a catheter is advanced into the right hepatic vein. A Colapinto needle (Cook Medical, Bloomington, IN, USA) is then used to access the portal vein from the right hepatic vein and iodinated contrast is injected (see **Fig. 1**C). In the setting of kidney failure or iodinated contrast allergy, venography can also be performed using carbon dioxide as a contrast agent.

PORTAL VEIN OCCLUSION ULTRASOUND IMAGING

Acute portal vein thrombosis causes either complete or partial occlusion of the portal vein.

The portal vein is typically well seen on ultrasound and nonvisualization of the portal vein is highly concerning for thrombosis. On grayscale imaging of acute complete portal vein occlusion, the thrombus is typically echo-poor and may be isoechoic or hypoechoic to the adjacent liver parenchyma, filling the entire portal vein (**Fig. 2**A). The vessel proximal to the thrombus is typically dilated and absence of flow can be confirmed by spectral and color Doppler (see **Fig. 2**A).

Grayscale imaging of partial thrombosis of the portal vein demonstrates isoechoic or hypoechoic thrombus eccentrically located along the vessel wall or floating within the vein (see **Fig. 2**B). Color

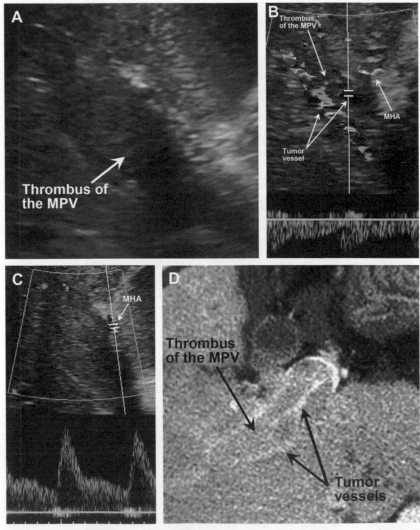

Fig. 4. Tumor thrombus. Ultrasound and CT imaging of main portal vein thrombus secondary to tumor invasion. (*A*) Grayscale images demonstrate an isoechoic thrombus of the main portal vein (MPV). (*B, C*) Color Doppler images within the portal vein thrombus show vascular flow with and arterial spectral waveform (*B*) highly concerning for a tumor vessel. A spectral tracing of the main hepatic artery (MHA) is also shown (*C*). (*D*) Contrast-enhanced CT shows arterial enhancing vessels within the main portal vein (MPV) thrombus consistent with tumor vascularity.

flow can be seen moving past the thrombus; however, the thrombus may sometimes be obscured by color bleed artifact. With minimally occlusive thrombus, color Doppler can demonstrate normal hepatopetal flow into the liver and a normal portal venous waveform is present on spectral Doppler in the patent portion of the vessel (see **Fig. 2**B). With severe partial thrombosis of the portal vein, elevated spectral velocities can be seen at the point of greatest stenosis and the stenosis may lead to upstream reversal of flow on color Doppler.

Transition to chronic portal vein thrombosis occurs when hepatopetal collateral veins begin to develop around the thrombosed portal vein, allowing blood to bypass the obstruction, leading to cavernous transformation of the porta hepatis. As the portal thrombus ages, the thrombus typically becomes more echogenic on grayscale imaging when compared with the background liver parenchyma and linear areas of calcification may occur within the thrombus (**Fig. 3**A). As with acute portal vein thrombosis, there is absence of flow in the

portal vein on color and spectral Doppler imaging (see **Fig. 3**A). On grayscale imaging, the diverting collateral vessels are seen as multiple anechoic tubular structures surrounding the thrombosed portal vein (see **Fig. 3**B). There is a mixed color pattern as the collateral vessels twist around the thrombosed portal vein with hepatopetal flow on color Doppler and spectral Doppler imaging demonstrates slow flow (see **Fig. 3**C).

Tumor thrombus is a unique form of portal vein thrombosis that occurs secondary to local tumor invasion into the portal vein. As with portal vein thrombosis secondary to clot, also known as bland thrombosis, tumor thrombosis is typically echo-poor and may be isoechoic or hypoechoic to the adjacent liver parenchyma (**Fig. 4**A). On color imaging, vascular flow is seen within the thrombus and demonstrates an arterial wave pattern on spectral Doppler imaging, corresponding to tumor vessel invasion (see **Fig. 4**B). A CT scan can be used to confirm the presence of tumor thrombus as manifested by contrast enhancement within the tumor vessels on arterial phase imaging

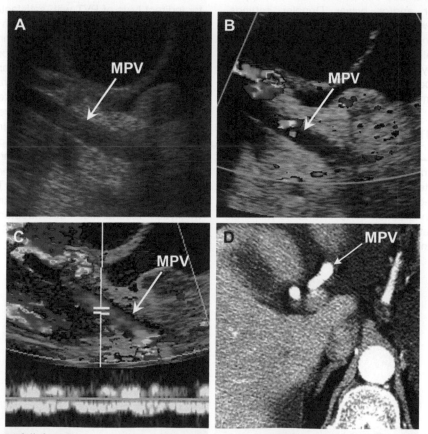

Fig. 5. Mimic: pitfall slow flow. Ultrasound and grayscale imaging of the main portal vein (MPV). Original grayscale (*A*) and color Doppler (*B*) imaging failed to demonstrate blood flow in the main portal vein. (*C*) Flow was then detected when the transducer frequency was lowered from 4 to 2.5 MHz and the wall filter was decreased to 55. (*D*) Contrast-enhanced CT confirmed the presence of portal vein flow.

and lack of portal enhancement on portal venous imaging (see **Fig. 4**D).

Slow portal flow is a pitfall of ultrasound imaging and can be a mimic of portal vein thrombosis if not recognized. Ultrasound cannot clearly detect portal vein flow if the velocity drops below 2 cm per second[5] and becomes even harder to evaluate when the portal vein is located deep within the patient. Lowering the transducer frequency, reducing the wall filter, switching to power Doppler, and lowering the velocity scale can all increase the detection of portal flow (**Fig. 5**). In addition, respiratory modulation may still be observed within the spectral waveform even when portal velocities drop below 2 cm per sec indicating the presence of portal flow.

Aliasing within the portal vein is a pearl of ultrasound imaging for the recognition of partial portal vein thrombosis. Because the main portal vein is a large to medium caliber vessel, regions of turbulent flow, which can be seen as aliasing on color Doppler, are not typically seen and may represent an obscured partial thrombus of the main portal vein. The thrombus can be revealed with appropriate color and/or power Doppler settings, including lowering the gain and/or lowering the wall filter. In addition, grayscale imaging in the region of aliasing can aid in the detection of thrombus by demonstrating a space filling isoechoic or hypoechoic structure outlined by residual anechoic lumen (**Fig. 6**).

TREATMENT OF PORTAL VEIN THROMBOSIS
Acute

Medical management is the first tool of choice in uncomplicated acute portal vein thrombosis, with complete recannulization in approximately 50%, partial recannulization in 40%, and no response in 10% of patients.[4,6] Patients are typically started on subcutaneous low molecular weight heparin and are then transitioned to vitamin K antagonists in 2 to 3 weeks with a target international normalized ratio of 2 to 3.[6] Recannulization of the portal vein is monitored with serial ultrasound imaging at 3 and 6 months as long as patient symptoms are improving (**Fig. 7**).[6] Interventional therapy is indicated in patients presenting with extensive thrombus of the portal vein, symptoms of progressive intestinal ischemia, ascites, and severe disease unresponsive to anticoagulation therapy.[4,6]

Transcatheter-directed thrombolysis allows for the local administration of a thrombolytic agent over a 6 to 48 hour period (**Fig. 8**). Agents of choice include urokinase at a concentration of 50,000–100,000 IU per hour or tissue plasminogen activator (tPA) at a concentration of 0.25 to 0.5 mg/hour. Using a transhepatic approach under fluoroscopic guidance, the portal vein is entered and an infusion catheter is placed along the length of the PVT. The small holes along the length of the catheter allow for a slow infusion of thrombolytic agent over the desired time period. If the portal vein is not accessible, the infusion catheter can also be placed intra-arterially within the superior mesenteric artery for indirect lysis of PVT with satisfactory results.[7] Depending on the extent of portal vein thrombosis, visualization of the portal vein may be limited fluoroscopically and intraoperative ultrasound can be used to both locate the portal vein and guide instrumentation placement. Overall, transcatheter-directed thrombolysis demonstrates superior reduction in thrombus burden and restoration of at least partial portal vein flow when compared with systemic thrombolytic therapy alone.[7]

Mechanical fragmentation of thrombosis is a more aggressive interventional technique for the treatment of portal vein thrombosis. Two devices are commonly used for this procedure. AngioJet rheolytic mechanical thrombectomy system (Possis Medical, Minneapolis, MN, USA) is a guidewire directed hydrodynamic apparatus that

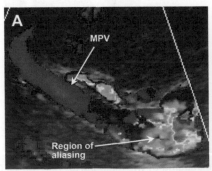
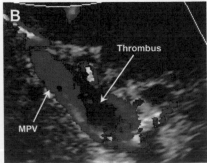

Fig. 6. Mimic: pearl aliasing. Color Doppler images of the main portal vein (MPV). (*A*) Original imaging of the main portal vein demonstrated a region of aliasing in the proximal main portal vein. (*B*) Reducing the gain revealed a partial thrombus in this region.

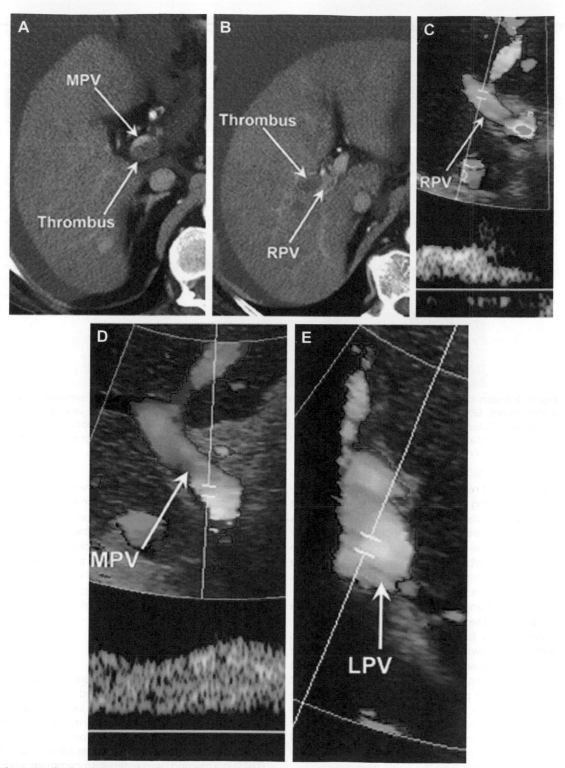

Fig. 7. Medical treatment of acute portal vein thrombosis. A case of acute portal vein thrombosis in the setting of cirrhotic liver morphology. (*A, B*) CT images obtained at clinical presentation involving different portal vein levels demonstrating extensive thrombus of the right and main portal vein (MPV) extending to the level of the confluence. (*C–E*) Ultrasound images obtained 4 months after anticoagulation therapy demonstrate complete resolution of portal vein thrombus, with unobstructed flow in the main (MPV), right (RPV), and left portal veins (LPV).

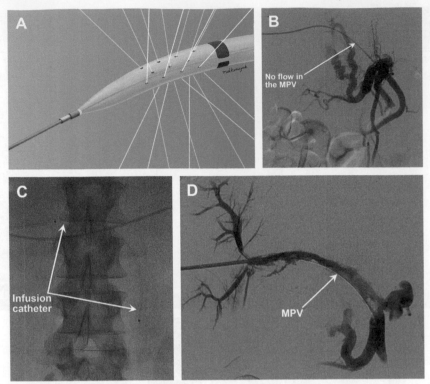

Fig. 8. Infusion catheter. (*A*) An infusion catheter. Images B–D demonstrate a case of failed systemic medical management. (*B*) Initial angiography demonstrated complete thrombus of the main portal vein (MPV) with extensive collateral formation. (*C*) An infusion catheter was placed along the thrombosed portal vein. (*D*) 48 hours of transcatheter-directed thrombolysis with tissue plasminogen activator (tPA) restored partial flow through the main (MPV) and right portal vein.

creates a fast retrograde fluid stream at the catheter tip causing a shear gradient to break up the thrombus. As the clot is destroyed, the fragments are removed through the lumen of the catheter (**Fig. 9**).[8,9] The Amplatz thrombectomy device (Microvena, White Bear Lake, MN, USA) has a high-speed impeller at the distal tip of the device, which creates a strong whirlpool within the thrombus, fragmenting the thrombus when it comes in contact with the impeller.[8,10]

Angioplasty is a mechanical technique used to widen a narrowed vessel (**Fig. 10**). Using a guide wire, a collapsed angioplasty balloon is placed at the site of obstruction. The balloon is then inflated to a fixed size under fluoroscopic imaging using water pressure. The expanding balloon crushes the clot circumferentially, increasing the caliber of the vessel lumen. The balloon is then deflated and either moved into another position for reinflation or removed along the guide wire.

Interventional treatment of acute portal vein thrombosis often uses a combination of multiple interventional techniques. At the authors' institution, medical management is attempted first unless poor prognostic indicators are present.

For those needing interventional therapy, we begin with local infusion of a thrombolytic agent for a period of 6 to 24 hours, following which the extent of recannulization is assessed. If the degree of recannulization is not adequate, mechanical removal of thrombus and/or angioplasty is then performed. Once interventional treatment is completed, the patient is placed back on medical therapy and the portal vein patency can be followed via ultrasound imaging.

CHRONIC

Interventional treatment of chronic portal vein thrombosis is typically requested secondary to symptoms of portal hypertension, including intractable ascites and variceal hemorrhage, and not usually to alleviate the portal thrombus itself.[4,11] Transjugular intrahepatic portosystemic shunt (TIPS) is a method used establish a communication between the hepatic vein and the portal vein (**Fig. 11**). This procedure requires the presence of patent intrahepatic portal branches; however, it can be accomplished with older thrombus and after cavernous transformation of the porta

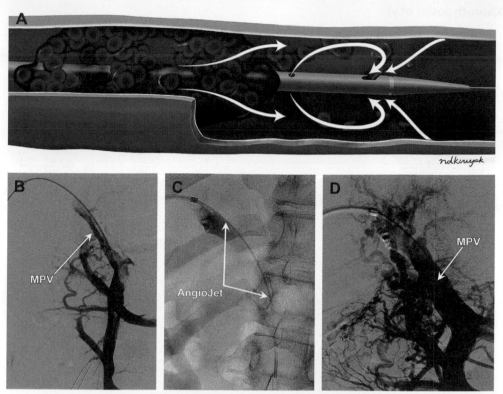

Fig. 9. Mechanical thrombectomy. (*A*) An AngioJet device. Images B–D demonstrate a case of symptomatic postoperative acute portal vein thrombosis with complete thrombus of the main portal vein (MPV) and extensive collateral formation. (*B*) After 24 hours of local transcatheter-directed thrombolysis, angiography reveals partial restoration of flow in the main portal vein. (*C*) AngioJet was then deployed along the length of the main portal vein. (*D*) Repeat angiography reveals significantly improved flow in the main portal vein.

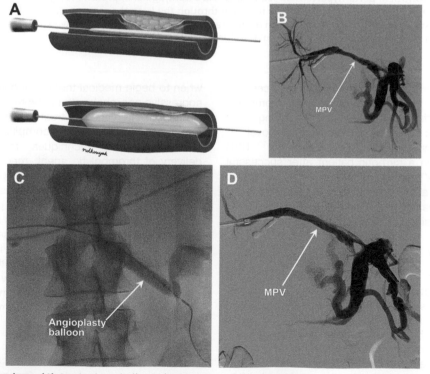

Fig. 10. Angioplasty. (*A*) Angioplasty balloon deployment within the vessel. Images B–D demonstrate the continuation of the case of failed systemic medical management depicted in **Fig. 8**. (*B*) Angiography demonstrates partial flow in the main portal vein (MPV) and right portal vein with no flow in the left portal vein. (*C*) An angioplasty balloon is deployed along the length of main portal vein thrombus. (*D*) Repeat angiography demonstrates improved flow within the main portal vein.

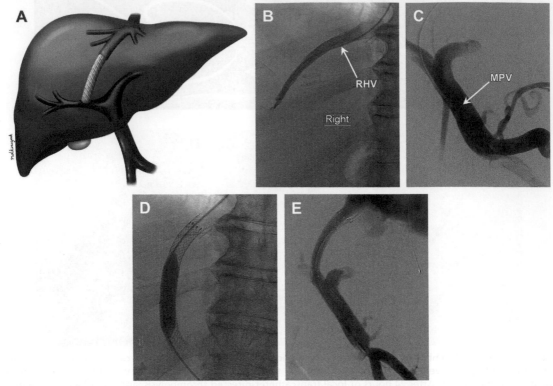

Fig. 11. Transjugular intrahepatic portosystemic shunt. (*A*) TIPS placement between the right hepatic vein and the right portal vein. Angiographic images B–E demonstrate TIPS placement in an individual with Laennec cirrhosis for symptomatic control of portal hypertension sequela. (*B*) Via a transjugular approach the right hepatic vein (RHV) is entered. (*C*) Using a curved Colapinto needle to pierce through the liver, the main portal vein (MPV) is entered. (*D*) Angioplasty is performed along the length of the tract and a covered stent is deployed. (*E*) Final angiography demonstrates a patent channel extending from the right portal vein to the right hepatic vein.

hepatis has occurred.[12] After shunt placement, transjugular treatment of portal vein thrombosis can be performed if requested, including local thrombolytic therapy, mechanical removal of thrombus, angioplasty, and/or stenting.[8,12] TIPS placement in a cirrhotic patient after successful or partial PVT treatment has also been performed to promote a high velocity flow through the portal vein, decreasing the risk of repeat thrombosis and decreasing the overall thrombus burden.[4,6]

SUMMARY

Thrombosis of the portal vein is a complicated medical entity that has a range of clinical symptoms from asymptomatic to life threatening. Ultrasound examination of the portal vein is the imaging modality of choice to initially evaluate for portal vein thrombosis, aid in intraprocedural instrumentation placement, and for the follow-up assessment of PVT therapy. Understanding the pearls and pitfalls of ultrasound imaging can help guide the clinical management of PVT, including the decision of

when to begin medical therapy and when a more aggressive approach with interventional radiology is needed. Interventional treatment of portal vein thrombosis is typically accomplished through a combination of techniques, including local delivery of thrombolytic agent, mechanical fragmentation of thrombus, and/or angioplasty. Treatment of chronic portal vein thrombosis with TIPS is typically directed at the symptoms of portal hypertension, including intractable ascites and variceal hemorrhage, with the possibility of secondary interventional treatment of PVT. Finally, in the setting of cirrhosis, TIPS may be subsequently used after PVT treatment to increase blood flow through the portal vein, thereby reducing thrombus burden and decreasing repeat thrombus formation.

ACKNOWLEDGMENTS

Images were created by Gwen Mack and Nadezhda Kiriyak, Department of Imaging Sciences, University of Rochester.

REFERENCES

1. Janssen H. Role of coagulation in the natural history and treatment of portal vein thrombosis. J Gastroenterol Hepatol 2001;16:595–6.
2. Sheen C, Lamparelli H, Milne A, et al. Clinical features, diagnosis and outcome of acute portal vein thrombosis. QJM 2000;93:531–4.
3. Webster G, Burroughs A, Riordan S. Review article: portal vein thrombosis—new insights into aetiology and management. Aliment Pharmacol Ther 2005;21(1):1–9.
4. Parikh S, Shah R, Kapoor P. Portal vein thrombosis. Am J Med 2010;123(2):111–9.
5. Görg C, Riera-Knorrenschild J, Dietrich J. Colour doppler ultrasound flow patterns in the portal venous system. Br J Radiol 2002;75:919–29.
6. Primignani M. Portal vein thrombosis, revisited. Dig Liver Dis 2010;42:163–70.
7. Thomas R, Ahmand S. Management of acute post-operative portal vein thrombosis. J Gastrointest Surg 2010;14:570–7.
8. Uflacker R. Applications of percutaneous mechanical thrombectomy in transjugular intrahepatic portosystemic shunt and portal vein thrombosis. Tech Vasc Interv Radiol 2003;6(1):59–69.
9. Stambo G, Grauer L. Transhepatic portal venous power-pulse spray rheolytic thrombectomy for acute portal vein thrombosis after CT-guided pancrease biopsy. AJR Am J Roentgenol 2005;184: S118–9.
10. Muller-Hulsbeck S, Hopfner M, Hilbert C, et al. Mechanical thrombectomy of acute thrombosis in transjugular intrahepatic portosystemic shunts. Invest Radiol 2000;35(6):385–91.
11. Tsochatzis E, Senzolo M, Germani G, et al. Systemic review: portal vein thrombosis in cirrhosis. Aliment Pharmacol Ther 2010;31:366–74.
12. Senzolo M, Tibbals J, Cholongitas E, et al. Transjugular intrahepatic portosystemic shunt for portal vein thrombosis with and without cavernous transformation. Aliment Pharmacol Ther 2006;23: 767–75.

REFERENCES

Hepatic Artery After Liver Transplant
Ultrasonographic Diagnosis for Intervention

Adam S. Fang, MD*, Ashwani K. Sharma, MD,
Deborah J. Rubens, MD

KEYWORDS

- Liver transplantation • Hepatic artery • Hepatic arterial complications • Hepatic artery thrombosis
- Hepatic artery stenosis • Hepatic artery pseudoaneurysm • Hepatic arteriovenous fistula

KEY POINTS

- Liver transplantation is the first-line treatment of acute and chronic end-stage liver diseases.
- Hepatic arterial complications limit the long-term success of the allograft.
- Early identification is crucial for graft salvage, and ultrasonography (US) is a valuable screening modality for the diagnosis of the most common and clinically significant complications, which include hepatic artery thrombosis, hepatic artery stenosis, hepatic artery pseudoaneurysm, and hepatic arteriovenous fistula.
- Understanding the unique clinical presentations, US findings, and therapeutic image-guided interventions of these complications can lead to early diagnosis and treatment to prevent graft failure and the need for retransplantation.

INTRODUCTION

Acute and chronic end-stage liver diseases have few successful therapeutic options, except for liver transplantation. Hepatic artery complications can occur and can lead to significant morbidity, mortality, and even retransplantation in the postoperative period. US is a valuable screening technique for the evaluation of early and delayed vascular complications and is often used as the initial imaging modality because of its accessibility, cost effectiveness, and noninvasive nature.[1–4]

ANATOMY AND POSTOPERATIVE NORMAL US FINDINGS OF HEPATIC ARTERY

A basic understanding of the variety of surgical techniques involved in liver transplantation is needed to identify the common postoperative complications. Heterotopic or orthotopic liver transplantation (OLT) can be performed using cadaveric whole-liver, reduced-size, split, or living donor liver transplants. The arterial anastomosis is performed using a branch patch technique, in which a fish-mouth anastomosis is made between the branch point of the donor common hepatic and splenic arteries and the origin of the recipient gastroduodenal artery from the common hepatic artery. Alternatively, a Carrel patch of the celiac axis and more complicated arterial reconstructions can be used for variant hepatic artery anatomy.[5–7] When there is high-grade stenosis in the native hepatic artery or celiac axis, an aortohepatic interposition graft of the donor iliac artery may be anastomosed to either the supraceliac or the infrarenal aorta.[7] The near-equal diameter

Disclosure: The authors do not have financial relationship with a commercial organization that may have a direct or indirect interest in the content.
Department of Imaging Sciences, University of Rochester Medical Center, 601 Elmwood Avenue, Box 648, Rochester, NY 14642, USA
* Corresponding author.
E-mail address: Adam_Fang@URMC.Rochester.edu

Ultrasound Clin 8 (2013) 249–258
http://dx.doi.org/10.1016/j.cult.2012.12.009
1556-858X/13/$ – see front matter © 2013 Elsevier Inc. All rights reserved.

ultrasound.theclinics.com

and lack of surplus vessel length of the donor and recipient vessels must be thoroughly evaluated to avoid potential vascular complications.

Postoperative evaluation of liver transplants involves gray scale, color Doppler, and duplex Doppler US focusing on the hepatic arteries, portal veins, hepatic veins, and inferior vena cava (IVC). Normal hepatic artery appearance is important for identifying hepatic arterial complications. The normal spectral Doppler waveform demonstrates a sharp systolic upstroke with continuous diastolic flow and a low-resistance waveform.[8] The normal resistive index (RI), defined as the difference between the peak systolic velocity and the peak diastolic velocity divided by the peak systolic velocity, is between 0.50 and 0.80 (**Fig. 1**A).[9] The RI is abnormal in patients with hepatic artery stenosis or hepatic artery thrombosis with collaterals (**Fig. 2**). An absent hepatic artery waveform or reflected pulsations (wall thump) indicates hepatic artery thrombosis (see **Fig.** 1B). During the first 72 hours after liver transplantation the RI may be increased, particularly in liver transplants with older donor age (>50 years old) or extended preservation.[9] Increased RIs may not be clinically significant if there is reported arterial flow and can be managed with serial ultrasound.[8,10] However, if there is any clinical suspicion of hepatic arterial complication, further evaluation with computed tomographic angiography, magnetic resonance angiography, or conventional angiography can be performed.[8,10]

HEPATIC ARTERY COMPLICATIONS

The major hepatic arterial complications include hepatic artery thrombosis, hepatic artery stenosis, hepatic artery pseudoaneurysm, and hepatic arteriovenous fistula.

Hepatic Artery Thrombosis

Background

The most significant and devastating postoperative complication after liver transplantation is hepatic artery thrombosis, which has a mortality rate of 33.3% (range 0%–80%) and requires urgent retransplantation in almost 50% of patients.[11–17] The entire donor biliary system is supplied by oxygenation from the hepatic artery. With loss of hepatic arterial perfusion, biliary stenosis or necrosis with bile stasis, abscess formation, and sepsis can occur. The incidence of hepatic artery thrombosis after liver transplantation is 4% to 11%,[5,12,14,18–22] and in the pediatric population, the incidence is 11% to 26%.[12,20–23] The most common risk factors for hepatic artery thrombosis include poor vascular conditions, increased blood flow resistance, small donor arteries, improper anastomosis, and rejection.[11,18,22–24] Hepatic artery thrombosis can be classified depending on the time of onset into early (during the first month after OLT) or late (≥1 month after OLT).[25] The incidence of early and late hepatic artery thromboses is between 33% to 46% and 1% to 25%, respectively.[26,27] Graft dysfunction usually does not occur because of formation of collateral blood supply. However, bile duct strictures, necrosis, bilomas, and abscess can still occur depending on the degree of biliary duct oxygenation. Symptoms and clinical presentation of hepatic artery thrombosis range from clinically asymptomatic to fulminant hepatic necrosis, delayed biliary leak, and relapsing bacteremia.[12,13,22]

Diagnosis on US

Given the occurrence of early hepatic artery thrombosis Doppler US surveillance is usually performed within the first 24 hours and frequently up to the time of discharge. The sensitivity of US in

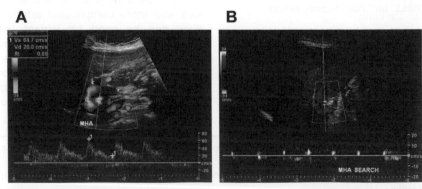

Fig. 1. (*A*) Normal hepatic artery. Duplex sonogram of the main hepatic artery (MHA) demonstrates sharp systolic upstroke and low-resistance waveform with a RI between 0.50 and 0.80. (*B*) Main hepatic artery thrombosis. Spectral tracing in the location of the main hepatic artery demonstrates no normal hepatic artery tracing, only reflected pulsations (wall thump) from the more proximal patent vessels. Vd, diastolic velocity; Vs, systolic velocity.

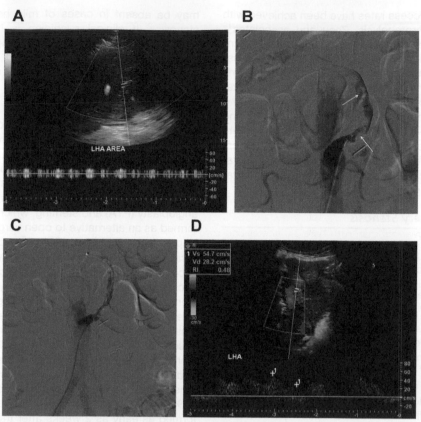

Fig. 2. Hepatic artery thrombosis. (*A*) Duplex sonogram of the left hepatic artery (LHA) in a patient with a jump graft demonstrates no arterial flow. (*B*) Digital subtraction angiographic image of the jump graft showed intraluminal filling defects (*arrows*) throughout the vessel. (*C*) Transcatheter thrombolysis was performed with tPA infusion for 24 hours and shows slight improvement, but the vessel is still not normal. (*D*) Follow-up duplex sonogram of the LHA confirms reestablishment of the hepatic artery flow; however, it is abnormal with a parvus–tardus waveform and low RI (<0.5) indicating either residual stenosis or collateral flow. Vd, diastolic velocity; Vs, systolic velocity.

diagnosing hepatic artery thrombosis is 92%.[28] On color and spectral Doppler US, there is absence of color and spectral Doppler flow within the hepatic artery (see **Fig. 2**A). If collateral flow is present, hepatic arterial tracings may exhibit an RI less than 0.5 and parvus–tardus waveforms, mimicking hepatic arterial stenosis. The microbubble contrast medium has been used successfully to improve the diagnostic capability of detecting acute hepatic artery thrombosis.[29]

Management

Revascularization is critical to prevent biliary ischemia and necrosis. Although the preferred treatment is thrombectomy with revision of the surgical anastomosis, most patients require retransplantation. However, the limited supply of donors and poor postoperative survival rates make endovascular treatment of hepatic artery thrombosis a more favorable alternative for emergent revascularization and salvage of the transplanted liver. Aortography is performed before

intervention to identify the arterial anatomy, especially if there is clinical concern for a narrowed celiac trunk of an aorta–hepatic graft. Selective microcatheterization and arteriography of the hepatic artery can be performed for better visualization of the hepatic artery anatomy. Angiographic findings including abrupt termination, filling defects, or nonvisualization of the hepatic artery support the diagnosis of thrombosis (see **Fig. 2**B). The catheter is advanced inside the visualized thrombus, and 1 to 3 mg of intra-arterial tissue plasminogen activator (tPA) is injected (see **Fig. 2**C). A continuous transcatheter thrombolysis is performed with tPA and heparin overnight. A second-look angiogram is obtained the next day to monitor the response to treatment and to see if the clot has dissolved and the peripheral hepatic artery branches are perfused. Other agents, such as urokinase (Abbokinase) and abciximab (ReoPro) can also be used. Additional balloon angioplasty and stenting can improve revascularization of residual stenosis.

Varying success rates have been achieved with attempted thrombolysis. Zhou and associates[19] found that continuous transcatheter arterial thrombolysis with urokinase (Abbokinase) was successful in revascularization in all 8 patients with early hepatic artery thrombosis (see **Fig. 2**D). However Sabri and colleagues[30] found that only 1 of 4 patients with late hepatic artery thrombosis and none of the 3 patients with early hepatic artery thrombosis achieved restoration of hepatic artery flow with thrombolysis. No significant postoperative complication was reported, including intra-abdominal or anastomotic bleeding.

Hepatic Artery Stenosis

Background
Hepatic artery stenosis is the second most common complication in patients after liver transplantation, occurring in 5% to 13% of transplant recipients.[1,22,31–36] The most common location of stenosis is at the anastomosis, and the most common causes include clamp injury, intimal injury from perfusion catheters during surgery, anastomotic ischemia from disrupted vasa vasorum, or rejection.[2,37] Hepatic artery stenosis can occur within days or within months to years after liver transplantation. One-third of the cases occur during the first month. The clinical presentation varies from an asymptomatic patient with mild increased liver function tests to one with acute liver failure and biliary complications.[38] Without proper treatment, major morbidity and mortality can result leading to further complications including hepatic artery thrombosis, ischemia, biliary stricture, sepsis, and graft loss.[20]

Diagnosis on US
Doppler US is the screening modality of choice to detect hepatic artery stenosis in liver transplant recipients. On gray scale images, a focal area of narrowing involving the hepatic artery may be observed. The spectral Doppler analysis often demonstrates a peak systolic velocity of greater than 200 to 300 cm/s at the anastomotic site, an RI less than 0.5, and a systolic acceleration time of 0.08 seconds or more (**Fig. 3**A, B). Doppler waveforms downstream from the stenosis usually demonstrate a parvus–tardus morphology indicating severe stenosis. Other findings, such as aliasing and turbulence just distal to the stenotic segment, also support the diagnosis.[37] However, the presence of a low RI or dampened arterial waveform is not specific for hepatic artery stenosis. Other conditions, such as severe aortoiliac atherosclerosis and hepatic artery thrombosis with intrahepatic collaterals, can have a similar presentation.[39] Doppler waveform abnormalities

may be absent in cases of mild hepatic artery stenosis.[2] If clinical suspicion is high despite a normal Doppler US, catheter angiography is considered the gold standard and can provide further confirmation in the setting of questionable US findings.

Management
Early detection of hepatic artery stenosis is crucial for appropriate treatment and salvage of the hepatic graft. Conventional treatment has included surgical revision or retransplantation. However, more minimally invasive endovascular procedures are available, such as percutaneous transluminal angioplasty (PTA) and stenting, which can be performed as an alternative to open surgical revision. Hepatic artery PTA is usually indicated for a solitary focal stenosis. The procedure involves selective microcatheterization of the hepatic artery with subsequent arteriography to identify the area of stenosis (see **Fig. 3**C). After crossing the hepatic artery, heparin is administered. Balloon angioplasty followed by one of the several types of vascular stents can be performed across the stenosis to reduce the risk of acute thrombosis and/or dissection (see **Fig. 3**D). Successful percutaneous hepatic artery angioplasty occurs in up to 81% to 93%,[30,40–42] and stenting can be performed as early as 2 weeks after transplantation. The mean interval time from initial PTA to restenosis occurs later with stent placement (5.7 months) compared with angioplasty alone (2.7 months).[40] Potential complications include rupture and dissection, which varies between 7% and 9.5%. Hepatic artery thrombosis occurs at the rate of 5% at 30 days and 19% at 1 year.[40,41] Doppler US is recommended within the immediate period after angioplasty. The surveillance protocol after angioplasty includes immediate 1-week Doppler US followed by monthly US for at least 6 months.

Hepatic Artery Pseudoaneurysm

Background
Hepatic artery pseudoaneurysm is a rare complication after liver transplantation occurring in about 0.6% to 2% of patients and usually within the first few months posttransplant.[22,33,43,44] Patients may be asymptomatic or present clinically with acute shock from a ruptured pseudoaneurysm. Some patients experience hemobilia or upper gastrointestinal bleeding secondary to fistula formation between the aneurysm and the biliary tract or bowel. Hepatic artery pseudoaneurysms can be classified into intrahepatic or extrahepatic pseudoaneurysms, which differ in their etiologic, clinical, and radiologic characteristics. Intrahepatic pseudoaneurysms are commonly related to biliary

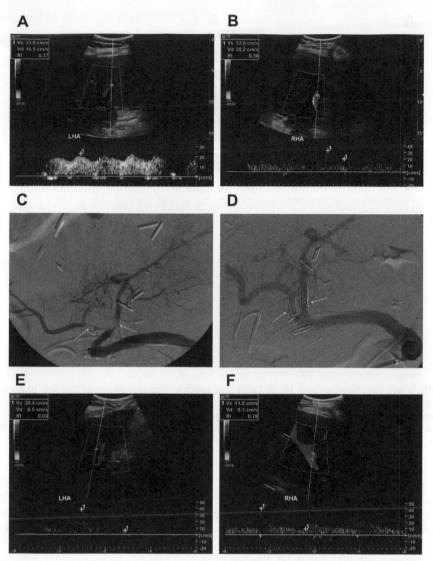

Fig. 3. Hepatic artery stenosis. (*A, B*) Duplex sonogram of the left hepatic artery (LHA) and right hepatic artery (RHA) in a patient with a jump graft demonstrates low-resistive waveforms with RI less than 0.5 and systolic acceleration time greater than 0.1 second suggesting significant left and right hepatic artery stenosis. (*C*) Digital subtraction angiographic (DSA) image from a selective microcatheterization of the patient's infrarenal jump graft confirms stenosis of the proximal LHA and RHA (*arrows*) distal to the graft. (*D*) DSA image postangioplasty and stenting (*arrows*) demonstrates successful treatment, with normal LHA and RHA waveforms on duplex sonogram (*E, F*). Vd, diastolic velocity; Vs, systolic velocity.

interventions, such as biopsy or biliary procedures. Extrahepatic pseudoaneursyms are often secondary to mycotic infections, such as fungal septicemia, and usually occur near the anastomotic site.[43]

Diagnosis on US

Nonthrombosed hepatic artery pseudoaneurysms appear as blind-ending cystic structures arising from the hepatic artery on gray scale Doppler US (**Fig. 4**A). Spectral Doppler analysis demonstrates disorganized waveform in the neck and a "to-and-fro" waveform within the lumen of the pseudoaneurysm with the "to" component occurring during systole and the "fro" component occurring during diastole (see **Fig. 4**B). On color Doppler, there is bidirectional color flow characteristically appearing as a "yin-yang" sign due to flow into and out of the pseudoaneurysm during each cardiac cycle.[43,44] A thrombosed hepatic artery pseudoaneurysm may be difficult to differentiate from postoperative hematoma.[43]

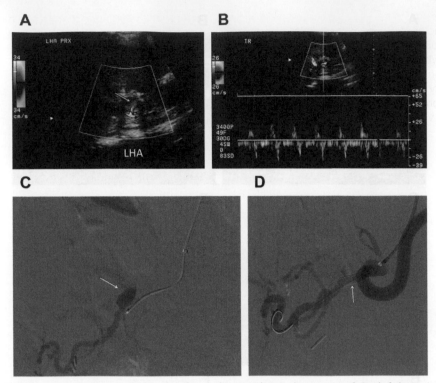

Fig. 4. Hepatic artery pseudoaneurysm. (*A, B*) Color and spectral Doppler image of the left hepatic artery (LHA) shows a blind-ending vascular structure with "to-and-fro" waveform (*arrow*), consistent with a pseudoaneurysm. (*C*) In a different patient, digital subtraction angiographic image from a selective microcatheterization of the patient's LHA shows a pseudoaneurysm (*arrow*). (*D*) Successful stent placement (*arrow*) excludes the pseudoaneurysm and is no longer patent.

Management

Given the risk of rupture, all hepatic artery pseudoaneurysms should be monitored and/or treated. Asymptomatic, small, and nonenlarging intrahepatic pseudoaneurysms can be managed conservatively with observation and follow-up imaging. However, symptomatic, large, or enlarging intrahepatic pseudoaneurysms require procedural intervention, such as surgical ligation of the involved intrahepatic artery, transplant segmentectomy, or even retransplantation. More minimally invasive procedures such as transcatheter or percutaneous embolization can also be performed with varying embolic agents including coils, Gelfoam (Pharmacia & Upjohn Company LLC, Cincinnati, OH, USA), thrombin, or detachable balloons. Transcatheter embolization typically uses coils to pack the hepatic artery pseudoaneurysm while maintaining downstream hepatic arterial perfusion. Percutaneous management can be guided with real-time US imaging.[45] The pseudoaneurysm can be accessed with a needle, following which coils or thrombin can be administered to obliterate the pseudoaneurysm. A balloon can be inflated at the neck of the hepatic

artery pseudoaneurysm during injection to prevent distal intrahepatic embolization. Extrahepatic pseudoaneursyms can be treated with surgical resection, embolization, or exclusion by stent placement (see **Fig. 4**C, D).

Hepatic Arteriovenous Fistula

Background

Hepatic arteriovenous fistulas are an uncommon complication after liver transplantation and can be classified into 2 types: arteriohepatic venous fistulas and arterioportal venous fistulas (APF). The latter are more common, occurring in 0% to 5.4% of abnormal liver transplant angiogram series.[22,46–48] The common causes of APF include needle biopsy, percutaneous transhepatic cholangiography, transhepatic catheterization of a portal vein, or fistualization of a mycotic aneurysm. Clinically, most APF are asymptomatic and most resolve spontaneously.[46,49,50] However, 17% of APF can be symptomatic,[46] leading to increased portal pressures and the development of esophageal varices, upper gastrointestinal tract bleeding, and ascites.[51,52]

Diagnosis on US

Color Doppler US is a valuable screening modality for the detection and diagnosis of APF.[53–61] When the velocity scale is set low, the fistulous communication may be identified by its high-velocity flow and the downstream arterialized waveform within the portal vein (**Fig. 5**A, B). The portal vein may also be dilated and show a poor response to the Valsalva maneuver on spectral Doppler analysis. The hepatic artery may have increased diastolic flow, resulting in an abnormally low resistance spectral Doppler tracing. Findings can be confirmed on arterial-phase computed tomography demonstrating early enhancement of the portal vein (see **Fig. 5**B).

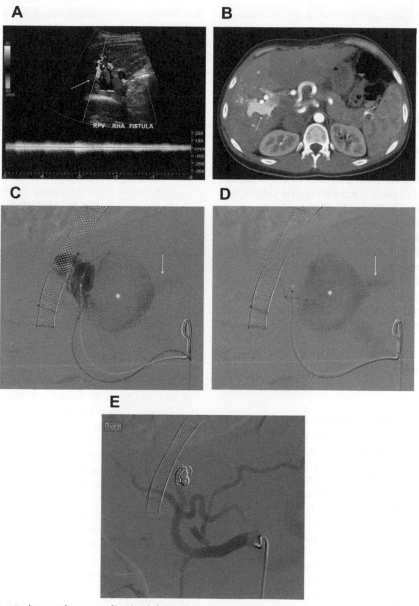

Fig. 5. Hepatic arterioportal venous fistula. (*A*) Duplex sonographic image demonstrates a right hepatic arterioportal venous fistula with high-velocity arterialized flow within the portal vein (*arrow*). (*B*) Arterial-phase CT shows early contrast enhancement of the right portal vein (*arrow*) confirming the diagnosis. (*C, D*) In a different patient, digital subtraction angiographic image from an early arterial injection of the right hepatic artery shows filling of an iatrogenic pseudoaneurysm (*asterisks*) created by prior transjugular intrahepatic portosystemic shunt procedure and portal vein (*arrows*) consistent with a hepatic arterioportal venous fistula. (*E*) Posttreatment with coiling demonstrates reduced flow through the fistula.

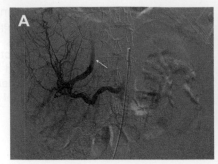
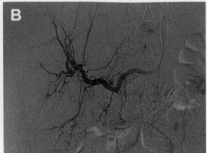

Fig. 6. Hepatic arteriohepatic venous fistula (*A*). Digitally subtracted angiogram (DSA) from a selective microcatheterization of the common hepatic artery shows shunting of blood from a branch of the left hepatic artery to the hepatic vein (*arrow*) consistent with an arteriohepatic venous fistula. (*B*) DSA image postembolization of the left hepatic artery with Gelfoam demonstrates successful treatment with absence of the shunt.

Management

In the past, APF were treated by surgical ligation, transplant segmentectomy, and retransplantation.[62–65] Recently, endoluminal embolization has emerged as an alternative management, particularly in patients with symptomatic APFs. Selective arteriography is performed with digital subtraction to identify the location of the fistula. A microcatheter is advanced to the fistula, and embolic agents such as, coils, Gelfoam (Pharmacia and Upjohn Company LLC, Cincinnati, OH, USA), or detachable balloons are deployed (see **Fig. 5**C, D; **Fig. 6**).[66,67] The goal is to reduce the shunting and prevent progression, which is not always possible. The most significant complication of embolization is hepatic artery thrombosis, which may result in graft loss.[50] The potential risk of hepatic artery thrombosis must be considered in all patients before attempting embolization.

SUMMARY

Liver transplantation is the first-line treatment of acute and chronic end-stage liver diseases. Hepatic arterial complications limit the long-term success of the allograft. Early identification is crucial for graft salvage, and US is a valuable screening modality for the diagnosis of the most common and clinically significant complications, which include hepatic artery thrombosis, hepatic artery stenosis, hepatic artery pseudoaneurysm, and hepatic arteriovenous fistula. Understanding the unique clinical presentations, US findings, and therapeutic image-guided interventions of these complications can lead to early diagnosis and treatment to prevent graft failure and the need for retransplantation.

REFERENCES

1. Garcia-Criado A, Gilabert R, Bargallo X, et al. Radiology in liver transplantation. Semin Ultrasound CT MR 2002;23:114–29.

2. Crossin JD, Muradali D, Wilson SR. US of liver transplants: normal and abnormal. Radiographics 2003; 23:1093–114.

3. Garcia-Criado A, Gilabert R, Nicolau C, et al. Early detection of hepatic artery thrombosis after liver transplantation by Doppler ultrasonography: prognostic implications. J Ultrasound Med 2001;20:51–8.

4. Ko EY, Kim TK, Kim PN, et al. Hepatic vein stenosis after living donor liver transplantation: evaluation with Doppler US. Radiology 2003;229:806–10.

5. Merion RM, Burtch GD, Ham JM, et al. The hepatic artery in liver transplantation. Transplantation 1989; 48:438–43.

6. Melada E, Maggi U, Rossi G, et al. Back-table arterial reconstructions in liver transplantation: single-center experience. Transplant Proc 2005;37(6): 2587–8.

7. Shaw BW, Iwatsuki S, Starzl TE. Alternative methods of arterialization of the hepatic graft. Surg Gynecol Obstet 1984;159(5):490–3.

8. Garcia-Criado A, Gilabert R, Berzigotti A, et al. Doppler ultrasound findings in the hepatic artery shortly after liver transplantation. AJR Am J Roentgenol 2009;193(1):128–35.

9. Brody MB, Rodgers SK, Horrow MM. Spectrum of normal or near-normal sonographic findings after orthotopic liver transplantation. Ultrasound Q 2008; 24(4):257–65.

10. Garcia-Criado A, Gilabert R, Salmeron JM, et al. Significance of and contributing factors for a high resistive index on Doppler of the hepatic artery immediately after surgery; prognostic implications for liver transplant recipients. AJR Am J Roentgenol 2003;181(3):831–8.

11. Stange BJ, Glanemann M, Nuessler NC, et al. Hepatic artery thrombosis after adult liver transplantation. Liver Transpl 2003;9(6):612–20.

12. Tzakis AG, Gordon RD, Shaw BW Jr, et al. Clinical presentation of hepatic artery thrombosis after liver transplantation in the cyclosporine era. Transplantation 1985;40(6):667–71.

13. Langnas AN, Marujo W, Stratta RJ, et al. Vascular complications after orthotopic liver transplantation. Am J Surg 1991;161(1):76–83.

14. Marujo WC, Langnas AN, Wood RP, et al. Vascular complications following orthotopic liver transplantation: outcome and the role of urgent revascularization. Transplant Proc 1991;23(1 Pt 2):1484–6.

15. Duffy JP, Hong JC, Farmer DG, et al. Vascular complications of orthotopic liver transplantation: experience in more than 4,200 patients. J Am Coll Surg 2009;208(5):896.

16. Bekker JS, Ploem S, de Jong KP. Early hepatic artery thrombosis after liver transplantation: a systematic review of the incidence, outcome, and risk factors. Am J Transplant 2009;9(4):746–57.

17. Singhal A, Stokes K, Sebastian A, et al. Endovascular treatment of hepatic artery thrombosis following liver transplantation. Transpl Int 2010;23(3): 245–56.

18. Oh CK, Pelletier SJ, Sawyer RG, et al. Uni- and multivariate analysis of risk factors for early and late hepatic artery thrombosis after liver transplantation. Transplantation 2001;71(6):767–72.

19. Zhou J, Fan J, Wang JH, et al. Continuous transcatheter arterial thrombolysis for early hepatic artery thrombosis after liver transplantation. Transplant Proc 2005;37(10):4426–9.

20. Blumhardt G, Ringe B, Lauchart W, et al. Vascular problems in liver transplantation. Transplant Proc 1987;19(1 Pt 3):2412.

21. Cheng YF, Chen YS, Huang TL, et al. Interventional radiologic procedures in liver transplantation. Transpl Int 2001;14(4):223–9.

22. Wozney P, Zajko AB, Bron KM, et al. Vascular complications after liver transplantation: a 5-year experience. AJR Am J Roentgenol 1986;147(4): 657–63.

23. Langnas A, Marujo W, Stratta RJ, et al. Hepatic allograft rescue following arterial thrombosis. Role of urgent revascularization. Transplantation 1991; 51(1):86–90.

24. Sanchez-Urdazpal L, Sterioff S, Janes C, et al. Increased bile duct complications in ABO incompatible liver transplant recipients. Transplant Proc 1991; 23(1 Pt 2):1440–1.

25. Bhattacharjya S, Gunson BK, Mirza DF, et al. Delayed hepatic artery thrombosis in adult orthotopic liver transplantation-a 12-year experience. Transplantation 2001;71(11):1592–6.

26. Ohdan H, Tashiro H, Ishiyama K, et al. Microsurgical hepatic artery reconstruction during living-donor liver transplantation by using head-mounted surgical binocular system. Transpl Int 2007;20(11): 970–3.

27. Gunsar F, Rolando N, Pastacaldi S, et al. Late hepatic artery thrombosis after orthotopic liver transplantation. Liver Transpl 2003;9(6):605–11.

28. Flint E, Sumkin J, Zajko A, et al. Duplex sonography of hepatic artery thrombosis after liver transplantation. AJR Am J Roentgenol 1988;151(3):481–3.

29. Grant EG, Melany M. Ultrasound contrast agents in the evaluation of the renal arteries. In: Goldberg BB, Raichlen JS, Forsberg F, editors. Ultrasound contrast agents. Basic principles and clinical applications. 2nd edition. London: Duntz; 2001. p. 289–95.

30. Sabri SS, Saad WE, Schmitt TM, et al. Endovascular therapy for hepatic artery stenosis and thrombosis following liver transplantation. Vasc Endovascular Surg 2011;45(5):447–52.

31. Quiroga S, Sebastia MC, Margarit C, et al. Complications of orthotopic liver transplantation: spectrum of findings with helical CT. Radiographics 2001; 21(5):1085–102.

32. Jain A, Costa G, Marsh W, et al. Thrombotic and nonthrombotic hepatic artery complications in adults and children following primary liver transplantation with long-term follow-up in 1000 consecutive patients. Transpl Int 2006;19(1):27–37.

33. Zajko AB, Campbell WL, Logsdon GA, et al. Cholangiographic findings in hepatic artery occlusion after liver transplantation. AJR Am J Roentgenol 1987; 149(3):485–9.

34. Orons PD, Sheng R, Zajko AB. Hepatic artery stenosis in liver transplant recipients: prevalence and cholangiographic appearance of associated biliary complications. AJR Am J Roentgenol 1995; 165(5):1145–9.

35. Saad WE. Management of hepatic artery steno-occlusive complications after liver transplantation. Tech Vasc Interv Radiol 2007;10(3):207–20.

36. Denys AL, Qanadli SD, Durand F, et al. Feasibility and effectiveness of using coronary stents in the treatment of hepatic artery stenosis after orthotopic liver transplantation: preliminary report. AJR Am J Roentgenol 2002;178(5):1175–9.

37. Dodd GD III, Memel DS, Zajko AB, et al. Hepatic artery stenosis and thrombosis in transplant recipients. Doppler diagnosis with resistive index and systolic acceleration time. Radiology 1994;192(3):657–61.

38. Dravid VS, Shapiro MJ, Needleman L, et al. Arterial abnormalities following orthotopic liver transplantation: arteriographic findings and correlation with Doppler sonographic findings. AJR Am J Roentgenol 1994;163(3):585–9.

39. Nghiem HV. Imaging of hepatic transplantation. Radiol Clin North Am 1998;36(2):429–43.

40. Saad WE, Davies MG, Sahler L, et al. Hepatic artery stenosis in liver transplant recipients: primary treatment with percutaneous transluminal angioplasty. J Vasc Interv Radiol 2005;16(6):795–805.

41. Orons PD, Zajko AB, Bron KM, et al. Hepatic artery angioplasty after liver transplantation: experience in 21 allografts. J Vasc Interv Radiol 1995;6(4):523–9.

42. Kodama Y, Sakuhara Y, Abo D, et al. Percutaneous transluminal angioplasty for hepatic artery stenosis after living donor liver transplantation. Liver Transpl 2006;12(3):465–9.

43. Marshall MM, Muiesan P, Kane PA, et al. Hepatic artery pseudoaneurysms following liver transplantation: incidence, presenting features and management. Clin Radiol 2001;56(7):579–87.

44. Stange B, Settmacher U, Glanemann M, et al. Aneurysms of the hepatic artery after liver transplantation. Transplant Proc 2000;32(3):533–4.

45. Patel JV, Weston MJ, Kessel DO, et al. Hepatic artery pseudoaneurysm after liver transplantation: treatment with percutaneous thrombin injection. Transplantation 2003;75(10):1755–7.

46. Saad WE, Davies MG, Rubens DJ, et al. Endoluminal management of arterio-portal fistulae in liver transplant recipients: a single center experience. Vasc Endovascular Surg 2006;40(6):451–9.

47. Karatzas T, Lykaki-Karatzas M, Webb M, et al. Vascular complications, treatment and outcome following orthotopic liver transplantation. Transplant Proc 1997;29(7):2853–5.

48. Zajko AB, Bron KM, Starzl TE, et al. Angiography of liver transplantation patients. Radiology 1985;157(2):305–11.

49. Okuda K, Musha H, Nakajima Y, et al. Frequency of intrahepatic arteriovenous fistulas as a sequela to percutaneous needle puncture of the liver. Gastroenterology 1978;74(6):1204–7.

50. Jabbour N, Reyes J, Zajko A, et al. Arterioportal fistula following liver biopsy. Three cases occurring in liver transplant recipients. Dig Dis Sci 1995;40(5):1041–4.

51. Vauthey JN, Tomczak RJ, Helmberger T, et al. The arterioportal fistula syndrome: clinicopathologic features, diagnosis, and therapy. Gastroenterology 1997;113(4):1390–401.

52. Pietri J, Remond A, Reix T, et al. Arterioportal fistulas: twelve cases. Ann Vasc Surg 1990;4(6):533–9.

53. Lumsden AB, Allen RC, Sreeram S, et al. Hepatic arterioportal fistula. Am Surg 1993;59(11):722–6.

54. Shapiro RS, Winsberg F, Stancato-Pasik A, et al. Color Doppler sonography of vascular malformations of the liver. J Ultrasound Med 1993;12(6):343–8.

55. Taourel P, Perney P, Bouvier Y, et al. Angiographic embolization of intrahepatic arterioportal fistula. Eur Radiol 1996;6(4):510–3.

56. Altuntas B, Erden A, Karakurt C, et al. Severe portal hypertension due to congenital hepatoportal arteriovenous fistula associated with intrahepatic portal vein aneurysm. J Clin Ultrasound 1998;26(7):357–60.

57. Tarazov PG, Prozorovskij KV. Intrahepatic spontaneous arterioportal fistula: duplex ultrasound diagnosis and angiographic treatment. Am J Gastroenterol 1991;86(6):775–8.

58. Lin ZY, Chang WY, Wang LY, et al. Clinical utility of pulsed Doppler in the detection of arterioportal shunting in patients with hepatocellular carcinoma. J Ultrasound Med 1992;11(6):269–73.

59. Mora P, Rabago L, Gea F, et al. Sonographic features of arterioportal fistula. J Clin Ultrasound 1992;20(4):291–3.

60. Tanaka S, Kitamura T, Fujita M, et al. Intrahepatic venous and portal venous aneurysms examined by color Doppler flow imaging. J Clin Ultrasound 1992;20(2):89–98.

61. Lafortune M, Breton G, Charlebois S. Arterioportal fistula demonstrated by pulsed Doppler ultrasonography. J Ultrasound Med 1986;5(2):105–6.

62. Hellekant C. Vascular complications following needle puncture of the liver. Clinical angiography. Acta Radiol Diagn 1976;17(2):209–22.

63. Chavan A, Harms J, Pichlmayr R, et al. Transcatheter coil occlusion of an intrahepatic arterioportal fistula in a transplanted liver. Bildgebung 1993;60(4):215–8.

64. Strodel WE, Eckhauser FE, Lemmer JH, et al. Presentation and perioperative management of arterioportal fistulas. Arch Surg 1987;122(5):563–71.

65. Agha FP, Raji MR. Successful transcatheter embolic control of significant arterioportal fistula: a serious complication of liver biopsy. Br J Radiol 1983;56(664):277–80.

66. Detry O, De Roover A, Delwaide J, et al. Selective coil occlusion of a large arterioportal fistula in a liver graft. Liver Transpl 2006;12(5):888–9.

67. Botelberge T, Van Vlierberghe H, Voet D, et al. Detachable balloon embolization of an arterioportal fistula following liver biopsy in a liver transplant recipient: a case report and review of the literature. Cardiovasc Intervent Radiol 2005;28(6):832–5.

Index

Note: Page numbers of article titles are in **boldface** type.

A

Ablation
    of tumors. *See* Tumor(s), ablation of.
    of varicose veins, 231–232
Abscess drainage, **117–124**
Achilles tenosynovitis, 198
Acromioclavicular joint
    cyst aspiration in, 194
    injections of, 193
Adenomyomas, uterine, focused ultrasound for,
    216–217
Amplatz thrombectomy device, for portal vein
    thrombosis, 244
Anesthesia, perivenous tumescent, for varicose vein
    treatment, 232
Angioplasty
    for hepatic artery stenosis, 252
    for portal vein thrombosis, 244–245
Ankle, interventions for, 198–199
Anticoagulants, for portal vein thrombosis, 242–243
Aortic dissection, percutaneous fenestration of,
    188–189
Arteriovenous fistulas, hepatic, after transplantation,
    254–256
Aspiration
    Baker cyst, 197
    breast cyst, 114
    fne-needle, for thyroid nodules, 155–160
    olecranon bursa, 194–195
    paralabral cyst, 194
    parameniscal cyst, 197
    scromioclavicular joint cyst, 194
    toe joints, 199
Automated systems, for breast lesions, 111–112
Axilla, lymph node biopsy in, 114–115

B

Bacteremia, in abscess drainage, 121
Baker cyst, aspiration of, 197
Balloon angioplasty
    for hepatic artery stenosis, 252
    for portal vein thrombosis, 244–245
Basilic vein, evaluation of, for hemodialysis access,
    139–140
Bethesda System for Reporting Thyroid
    Cytopathology, 157
Biceps tendonitis, 193–194
Biliary interventions, radiation reduction in, **165–170**

drainage, 166–169
    in cholecystostomy, 165–166
    in percutaneous transhepatic cholangiography,
        166–169
    real-time dosimetry in, 169–170
Biopsy
    breast, 113–114
    lymph nodes, 161–162, 207
    prostate, 207
    soft tissue, 161–162, 192
    solid organs, **147–154**
    thyroid, **155–163**
    ultrasound GPS for, 207
Biot Savart law, 203
BI-RAD (Breast Imaging Reporting and Data System),
    113
Bleeding
    after solid organ biopsy, 152–153
    in abscess drainage, 121
Bone, metastasis to, focused ultrasound for, 219
Bowel signature, in abscess drainage, 121–122
Brachial artery, evaluation of, for hemodialysis
    access, 138–139
Brachiocephalic vein, evaluation of, for hemodialysis
    access, 139
Brain tumors, focused ultrasound for, 222
Breast lesions, **109–116**
    automated technology for, 111–112
    axilla biopsy for, 114
    biopsy of, 113–114
    computer-aided diagnosis of, 112
    contrast-enhanced techniques for, 113
    cyst aspiration in, 114
    diagnosis of, 110, 112
    elastography for, 111
    focused ultrasound for, 219–221
    fusion imaging for, 112
    in dense breasts, 109–110
    screening for, 109–110
    second-look of, 110–111
    three-dimensional imaging for, 112–113
    wire localization for, 114

C

Calcific tendinopathy barbotage, 193
Cancer
    ablation of. *See* Tumor(s), ablation of.
    breast. *See* Breast lesions.

Ultrasound Clin 8 (2013) 259–264
http://dx.doi.org/10.1016/S1556-858X(13)00012-1
1556-858X/13/$ – see front matter © 2013 Elsevier Inc. All rights reserved.

Moving?

Make sure your subscription moves with you!

To notify us of your new address, find your **Clinics Account Number** (located on your mailing label above your name), and contact customer service at:

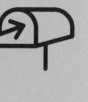

Email: journalscustomerservice-usa@elsevier.com

800-654-2452 (subscribers in the U.S. & Canada)
314-447-8871 (subscribers outside of the U.S. & Canada)

Fax number: 314-447-8029

Elsevier Health Sciences Division
Subscription Customer Service
3251 Riverport Lane
Maryland Heights, MO 63043

*To ensure uninterrupted delivery of your subscription, please notify us at least 4 weeks in advance of move.

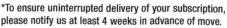

Printed and bound by CPI Group (UK) Ltd, Croydon, CR0 4YY

03/10/2024

01040346-0015